613.713 B1301f 2014
Baechle
Fitness
W9-AQA-222

# *FITNESS*
# *WEIGHT*
# *TRAINING*

## THIRD EDITION

**Thomas R. Baechle**
**Roger W. Earle**

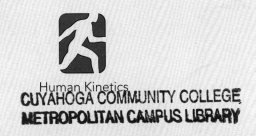

Human Kinetics

CUYAHOGA COMMUNITY COLLEGE
METROPOLITAN CAMPUS LIBRARY

**Library of Congress Cataloging-in-Publication Data**

Baechle, Thomas R., 1943-
 Fitness weight training / Thomas R. Baechle, Roger W. Earle. -- Third Edition.
   pages cm
 Includes index.
 1. Weight training. 2. Physical fitness. I. Earle, Roger W., 1967- II. Title.
 GV546.B33 2014
 613.7'13--dc23

                              2013049156

ISBN-10: 1-4504-4513-6 (print)
ISBN-13: 978-1-4504-4513-9 (print)

Copyright © 2014, 2005 by Thomas Baechle and Roger Earle
Copyright © 1995 by Human Kinetics, Inc.

All rights reserved. Except for use in a review, the reproduction or utilization of this work in any form or by any electronic, mechanical, or other means, now known or hereafter invented, including xerography, photocopying, and recording, and in any information storage and retrieval system, is forbidden without the written permission of the publisher.

This publication is written and published to provide accurate and authoritative information relevant to the subject matter presented. It is published and sold with the understanding that the author and publisher are not engaged in rendering legal, medical, or other professional services by reason of their authorship or publication of this work. If medical or other expert assistance is required, the services of a competent professional person should be sought.

Notice: Permission to reproduce the following material is granted to instructors and agencies who have purchased *Fitness Weight Training,* Third Edition: pp. 26, 27, and 247-253. The reproduction of other parts of this book is expressly forbidden by the above copyright notice. Persons or agencies who have not purchased *Fitness Weight Training,* Third Edition may not reproduce any material.

The web addresses cited in this text were current as of December 2013, unless otherwise noted.

**Acquisitions Editor:** Justin Klug; **Managing Editor:** Amy Stahl; **Assistant Editor:** Elizabeth Evans; **Copyeditor:** Jan Feeney; **Indexer:** Bobbi Swanson; **Permissions Manager:** Martha Gullo; **Graphic Designer:** Nancy Rasmus; **Graphic Artist:** Tara Welsch; **Cover Designer:** Keith Blomberg; **Photographs (cover and interior):** © Human Kinetics; **Visual Production Assistant:** Joyce Brumfield; **Photo Production Manager:** Jason Allen; **Art Manager:** Kelly Hendren; **Associate Art Manager:** Alan L. Wilborn; **Illustrations:** © Human Kinetics; **Printer:** United Graphics

We thank The Fitness Center Body Shop in Champaign, Illinois, for assistance in providing the location for the photo shoot for this book.

Human Kinetics books are available at special discounts for bulk purchase. Special editions or book excerpts can also be created to specification. For details, contact the Special Sales Manager at Human Kinetics.

Printed in the United States of America          10   9   8   7   6   5   4   3   2   1

The paper in this book is certified under a sustainable forestry program.

**Human Kinetics**
Website: www.HumanKinetics.com

*United States:* Human Kinetics
P.O. Box 5076
Champaign, IL 61825-5076
800-747-4457
e-mail: humank@hkusa.com

*Canada:* Human Kinetics
475 Devonshire Road Unit 100
Windsor, ON N8Y 2L5
800-465-7301 (in Canada only)
e-mail: info@hkcanada.com

*Europe:* Human Kinetics
107 Bradford Road
Stanningley
Leeds LS28 6AT, United Kingdom
+44 (0) 113 255 5665
e-mail: hk@hkeurope.com

*Australia:* Human Kinetics
57A Price Avenue
Lower Mitcham, South Australia 5062
08 8372 0999
e-mail: info@hkaustralia.com

*New Zealand:* Human Kinetics
P.O. Box 80
Torrens Park, South Australia 5062
0800 222 062
e-mail: info@hknewzealand.com

E5897

# FITNESS
# WEIGHT
# TRAINING

THIRD EDITION

# Contents

# Preface

In this section of earlier editions of *Fitness Weight Training*, we expressed the desire for a book that would make the greatest contribution to helping people experience the enjoyment and benefits of weight training. Since the first edition was published, *Fitness Weight Training* has sold over 125,000 copies and has been translated into five languages. Writing this third edition provided us with an opportunity to introduce new training options that have the potential to make even greater improvements in the quality of life for those who use this book.

Many times, we have discovered that one of the largest road blocks a person experiences when beginning a weight training program is simply not knowing what type of program to follow. For anyone who sets foot in a fitness facility, high school or college weight room, or even the sporting goods department of a retail store, seeing the many types of machines and equipment can be instantly intimidating. Even if the array of equipment is not overwhelming, figuring out how many sets and repetitions to perform and how much weight to lift can be.

This book will help you break through these barriers by providing you with

- a method that allows you to determine your initial weight training fitness level;
- information and questions to help you set a specific exercise goal;
- photographs and technique guidelines for 63 weight training exercises;
- information that will help in selecting the right equipment to use;
- step-by-step instructions for selecting your exercises and determining how much weight to lift; and
- 75 weight training programs arranged in six progressive workout zones that are geared for three unique exercise goals.

If you are already weight training, this book presents guidelines for cross-training with other types of exercise (like walking, running, biking, or swimming), upgrading your current program (or one found in this book) to improve your performance in sports and recreational activities, and the ultimate task of designing your own program from scratch.

# Acknowledgments

Special people in our lives support us and give us energy, and their love makes completing tasks, such as working on this book, easier. We dedicate this third edition of *Fitness Weight Training* to those special people:

Family members: Tom's wife, Susie; sons, Todd and Clark; and daughter-in-law, Orenda.

Roger's wife, Tonya, and daughters Kelsey, Allison, Natalia, and Cassandra.

HK staff: Justin Klug, Amy Stahl, Neil Bernstein, Joyce Brumfield, Jason Allen, Gregg Henness, Kelly Hendren, Nancy Rasmus, and Tara Welsch.

Photo shoot models: Amanda Hunter, Richard Hunter, Tiffany Meyer, Kyle Olsen, and Jennifer Rapp.

# Part I

# Prepare to Weight Train

Weight training is taking fitness enthusiasts by storm, and it has even become attractive to thousands who once called themselves couch potatoes. Weight training is an activity that you can accomplish in a short time, yet it can dramatically change how your body looks and feels. Many who weight train will tell you that having a firm body not only feels great but also positively affects how they relate to others. Following a regular program will increase your energy level and improve your productivity at work and in many everyday activities. Additional benefits include improving muscle strength, muscular endurance, neuromuscular (nerve–muscle) coordination, and bone density (helping to prevent osteoporosis). Weight training helps to prevent and manage type 2 diabetes and enhance cardiovascular health by lowering blood pressure and having a positive effect on controlling cholesterol and lipoprotein levels.

The latest research suggests that weight training also contributes significantly to quality of life, whatever one's sex or age. In fact, interest in weight training has increased considerably, especially among seniors.

No matter what your weight training experience is or what equipment you have access to, you will find helpful information in this book. If you have little or no experience in weight training, we provide the basics to get you started. If you have trained before but without much organization to your approach, you will benefit from the guidance offered by the structured programs. If you have a great deal of weight training experience, we will show you how to train better and get more from your workouts. Finally, if you want to weight train to improve performance in your favorite sport, this book describes how to develop a specific program that focuses on that outcome.

Part I begins by describing three types of training outcomes, which form the basis of the workouts in part II. The chapters in part I lay the groundwork for your weight training program by helping you to

- understand how the physical benefits of weight training compare with other activities;

- determine what weight training equipment to use, where to train, and how to choose and buy equipment;
- determine your weight training fitness level;
- choose your weight training goal;
- train safely and effectively; and
- set up your actual weight training program.

After you have identified your training goal and the appropriate workout zone, you will probably be eager to begin your new weight training program. Before jumping in to your first workout, however, be sure that you carefully consider all the guidelines, recommendations, and safety issues explained in this part of the book. Doing so will not only increase the probability of reaching your exercise goals but also reduce your risk of injury.

Let's get started!

# Weight Train to Improve Fitness

When we were asked to write the third edition of this book, we saw it as an opportunity to more clearly describe the benefits of weight training, add exercises, update photos, and streamline workouts. The no-nonsense approach has been retained and is complemented by the use of colors to designate training intensities, or zones. Our unique method of organizing and presenting workouts will enable you to begin weight training immediately, regardless of your fitness status. There are six levels of training intensity detailed in chapters 7 to 12; the workouts range from short and easy sessions for beginners to longer and intense sessions for the highly trained. Best of all, *Fitness Weight Training* enables you to match your goal to one of three training programs—muscle toning (to firm up your muscles), body shaping (to develop larger muscles), and strength training (to make you stronger)—and then provides you with a program for reaching your desired goal.

## Principle of Specificity

A well-designed weight training program is based on the principle of *specificity*—the crucial factor in any exercise program. Simply put, if you want to achieve a specific result, you need to design and then follow a specific training program. For example, the muscle toning program will cause your body to become more toned. Furthermore, when you select an exercise for each muscle group or body area, you apply the principle of specificity: to train the chest muscles, you choose a chest exercise, not a leg exercise, for instance.

The principle of specificity is important to incorporate into your program if you are training to improve your sport performance. Exercises should mimic the movement patterns that occur in your sport. For example, if you are a basketball player, you understand the importance of jumping. To apply the principle of specificity, you need to select weight training exercises that are similar to jumping so that your jumping ability will improve. Therefore, you would choose to perform the squat exercise rather than the leg extension or leg curl exercise. Although the leg extension and leg curl exercises train the leg muscles involved in jumping, the squat exercise more closely mimics the actual jumping motion.

## Muscle Toning

Toned muscles appear firm rather than flabby. They are also defined, which means that you can see distinct muscle separations, indentations, and shapes.

Muscle toning is a natural outcome of regular weight training. If you are interested in muscle toning, higher repetitions in your training will produce better muscle tone without large increases in muscle size. Therefore, the result of following a muscle toning program will be firmer and more defined muscles without significant increases in muscle size (figure 1.1).

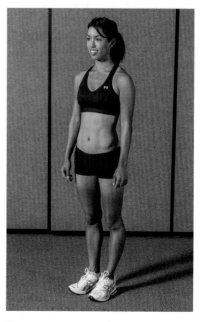

**Figure 1.1**  A muscle-toned woman.

## Body Shaping

Body shaping programs provide all the benefits associated with muscle toning programs, but they also increase the size of muscles more dramatically (figure 1.2). With body shaping, you will not only experience the muscle firming and definition of muscle toning but also increase your muscle size. This result is especially true for men; the physique of a woman who is weight training does not change as dramatically. Some women, however, may notice small changes in girth in the shoulders, thighs, arms, or back from a body shaping program.

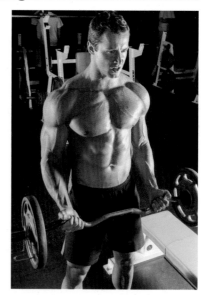

**Figure 1.2**  A body-shaped man.

# Strength Training

Strength is the ability of the muscle to exert force. Typically, the term *strength* is associated with the ability to exert maximum force during a single effort, sometimes referred to as a *one-repetition maximum* effort (1RM). For instance, someone gives you a weight of 100 pounds (45 kg) and then asks you to perform as many repetitions as possible (with proper technique) in the bench press exercise. If you could do only one repetition, your one-repetition maximum, or 1RM, would be 100 pounds. Increased strength can significantly improve performance in recreational and competitive sports as well as make everyday tasks—regardless of your age—much easier. A strength training program usually produces gains in muscle size that are greater than those achieved in a muscle toning program but not to the same degree as a body shaping program. (See figure 1.3.)

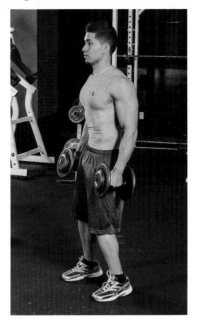

**Figure 1.3** A strength-trained man.

# Why Not Walk or Jog Instead?

Aerobic exercises such as walking and jogging are ideal for improving the fitness of your heart and lungs and the muscular endurance of your legs, but these activities contribute less to shaping your body and improving your overall flexibility, muscular endurance, and upper-body strength. The advantage of aerobic activities over weight training is that they require minimal equipment and can be done almost anywhere. Swimming, cycling, and cross-country skiing, which are also aerobic activities, are better than walking or jogging in terms of building overall flexibility, muscular endurance, and strength, but they still fall short of what weight training programs do for strengthening and shaping specific areas of the body. Weight training programs are more effective than aerobic programs in improving muscular strength, muscular endurance, body composition (ratio of muscle to fat), and flexibility.

For older adults who are inactive, weight training can be an especially important activity because muscle mass declines 5 to 10 percent each decade after age 50. This loss of muscle results in a decline in strength, which is often associated with a variety of illnesses, injuries, and infirmities. Research has demonstrated that younger as well as older adults who follow at least a 6-week weight training program will have significant increases in muscle mass and strength. Similar research has shown that weight training can also lower blood pressure, improve bone mineral density, and help people with diabetes improve insulin resistance and glucose tolerance.

Unlike other exercise activities that develop a limited number of muscles (for example, walking and cycling primarily develop the legs), weight training programs can help you develop many muscle groups—especially those that are particularly important to you. Weight training is like going through a cafeteria and picking which foods you want to eat instead of having to eat simply what is served to you. The workouts in chapters 7 through 12 emphasize exercises for seven major muscle groups: chest, back, shoulders, front of the arms, back of the arms, core, and legs. (See figure 1.4.) The workouts also condition the smaller muscles of the forearms, calves, and neck.

How well your program is designed and how diligently you follow it will determine your success in achieving your desired outcome. What makes weight training exciting is the rapid rate at which you can see and feel changes in your body. As soon as you start exercising, your muscles feel firmer, and the body sculpting process begins. Regular training will convince you that you have the ability to develop your body in ways that you may never have expected!

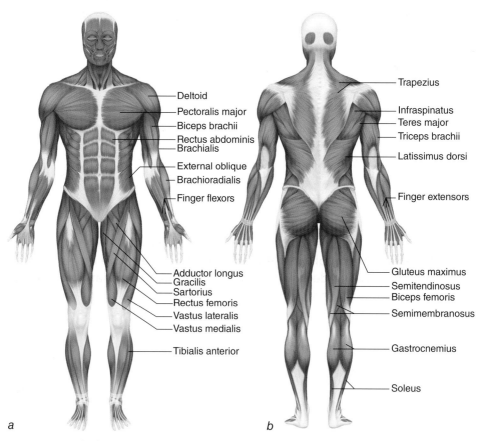

**Figure 1.4**   The body's major muscle groups: *(a)* front view; *(b)* rear view.

# Know Your Equipment and Understand Its Proper Use

Choosing your equipment and clothing and identifying a suitable place to train and qualified people to teach you are important considerations for weight training. This chapter informs you in all these areas so that you can get equipped with confidence! Keep in mind, though, that various types of weight training equipment (especially machines) may have a similar look but feel completely different when you use them.

## Types of Weight Training Equipment

Nearly all weight training exercises involve using machines, free weights (including barbells, dumbbells, and kettlebells), resistance bands, stability balls, or combinations of all of these. Machines and free weights are commonly seen in schools, health clubs, and corporate settings, whereas dumbbells, resistance bands, and stability balls are common in the home. Machines are less common in homes because they are expensive and require more space (although collapsible machines that save space are available). The following sections describe the types of equipment that you can use for performing the exercises in your program.

### Machines

Machine exercises require you to sit on, recline in, or stand next to the apparatus. You then move a part of the machine (such as a handle or bar attached to a chain or cable) to lift a weight rather than the weight itself. The two most common types of weight training machines are cam and pulley machines.

### Cam Machines

A cam machine is a variable-resistance machine that features an elliptically shaped wheel, referred to as a *cam*. As the chain, cable, or belt tracks over the peaks and valleys of the cam, the distance between the point of rotation (the axle on which the cam rotates) and the weight stack varies to produce a more consistent load on the muscles. An example of a cam machine is shown in figure 2.1.

### Pulley Machines

Many machines have one or more round pulleys of varying sizes (much smaller than a cam) looped around, over, or under by a narrow belt or plastic-encased steel cable. If the machine has one pulley, it only serves to change the direction that the weight stack moves compared to the direction you pull or push to move the weight stack (for example, when performing the low-pulley curl exercise, you pull up on the bar and the weight stack moves up). Machines designed with two or more pulleys offer a trade-off between the effort needed to move the weight stack and the distance (and, sometimes, the direction) that you have to pull or push to move the weight stack. One advantage is that you can train your muscles through a full range of motion and the weight stack only to move only a portion of that distance. An example of a pulley machine is shown in figure 2.2.

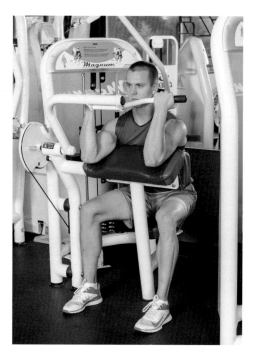

**Figure 2.1**   A cam machine.

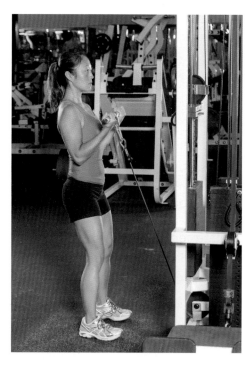

**Figure 2.2**   A pulley machine.

## Safety Considerations for Machines

Many consider training on machines to be safer than doing so with barbells and dumbbells because the weight stack is positioned and contained so that it cannot fall off or fall on the user. In addition, machine exercises typically do not require the same degree of muscular coordination needed for using barbells or dumbbells. Another advantage of machines is that you can perform exercises without a spotter. With that said, do not assume that you cannot be seriously injured on a machine. By understanding how to use machines properly (as discussed in chapter 5), you will find them to be a safe and time-efficient type of weight training equipment.

## Free Weights

Barbell, dumbbell, and kettlebell exercises are categorized as free weights. An exercise using free weights allows more freedom to move the weight in nearly any desired direction because you are actually holding the bar, dumbbell, or weight. Free-weight equipment costs less than weight machines and offers tremendous versatility, making your choice of exercises virtually unlimited.

### Barbells

Most two-arm and two-leg exercises involve a barbell. The typical barbell has a middle section that includes both smooth and *knurled* (roughened) areas with *collars* on each side. The weight plates slide up to collars that stop the plates from sliding inward toward the hands. The outside collars, sometimes referred to as *locks*, slide up and tighten next to the plates and keep them from sliding off the ends of the bar. A 6-foot (183 cm) bar with collars and locks weighs approximately 30 pounds (14 kg), or 5 pounds per foot (about 8 kg per meter) of the bar. *Cambered,* or curl, bars have the same characteristics as standard bars except that the curves enable you to isolate certain muscle groups better than you can when using a straight bar.

At many fitness facilities you will find 6-foot (183 cm) standard and cambered bars and 7-foot (213 cm) Olympic bars. Olympic bars have the same diameter as most bars except that the diameter is greater in the section between the collar and the end of the bar. Olympic bars are heavier than standard bars; they weigh 45 pounds (20 kg) without locks. Olympic-style weight plates, which have larger holes than standard weight plates, are designed for use only with Olympic bars. Barbell equipment is shown in figure 2.3.

### Dumbbells

Dumbbells are used in one- and two-arm exercises. Although they are some-times *premolded* (all one piece, without weight plates), some fitness facili-ties have dumbbells that have a design similar to barbells but with smaller weight plates. Dumbbells are much shorter than barbells, and the entire middle section (between the weight plates) is usually knurled. A dumbbell bar with collars and locks weighs approximately 3 pounds (1.4 kg). Usually only the weight of the plates is considered when the weight of the dumbbell is marked on the side of the outermost plate. For example, a dumbbell with a 10-pound plate on both sides is marked as weighing 20, not 23, pounds. Dumbbell equipment is also shown in figure 2.3.

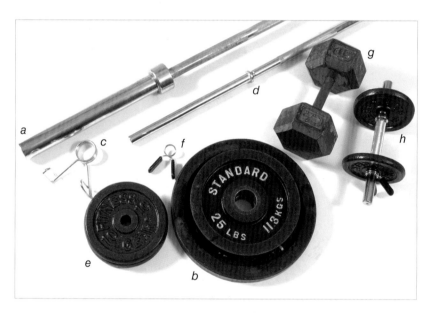

**Figure 2.3** Barbell and dumbbell equipment: *(a)* Olympic bar; *(b)* Olympic-style weight plate; *(c)* Olympic bar lock; *(d)* standard bar; *(e)* standard weight plate; *(f)* standard lock; *(g)* premolded dumbbell; *(h)* plate-loaded dumbbell.

### Kettlebells

A kettlebell resembles a cast-iron ball (like a cannonball) with a handle attached to the top of it. It can weigh as little as 9 pounds (4 kg) or more than 100 pounds (45 kg). It is different from a dumbbell because the weight of a kettlebell is distributed unevenly so your body has to work harder to maintain balance. You can do standard weight training exercises with kettle-bells, such as the double bent-over row and front squat (see chapter 6), but one advantage of using kettlebells is that they allow you to train multiple muscle groups at the same time and force those muscle groups to work together. The result is an excellent whole-body workout. An example of several kettlebells is shown in figure 2.4.

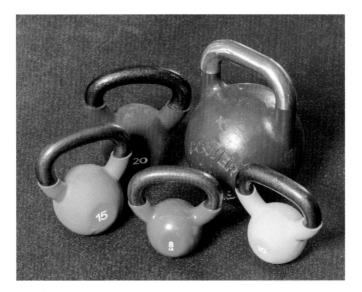

**Figure 2.4** Standard kettlebells.

## Safety Considerations for Free Weights

The term *free* in free weight means that the equipment does not restrict joint movement. Consequently, using free-weight barbells, dumbbells, and kettlebells requires a higher level of muscle coordination than using machines. Because of this freedom of movement, injuries are more likely to occur if you do not use correct loading, lifting, and spotting techniques. Plus, be sure you have enough space around and above you, especially when you are performing an overhead exercise or an exercise involving swinging or rotating with a kettlebell. When you take reasonable precautions (as discussed in chapter 5), free-weight training is safe and can be more fun than training with machines, and it is also more effective in strengthening joint structures.

## Resistance Bands

An alternative to a machine or free-weight exercise is one that uses a rubber tube or elastic cable to create resistance (figure 2.5). For example, instead of lifting a bar to perform the biceps curl, you can use a resistance band (see chapter 6).

Exercising with resistance bands is a convenient and practical choice if you cannot go to a fitness facility, have limited space at home, or travel frequently. Resistance bands come in various lengths, handle types, and colors, which indicate the relative degree of elasticity (see chapter 4 for more details).

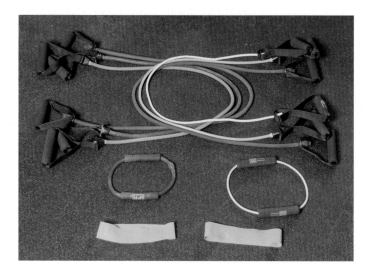

**Figure 2.5**   Various types of resistance bands.

## Safety Considerations for Resistance Bands

Beware of old, worn, or cracked bands that may break at the worst moment when you are using them. Also, check that the handles are securely attached to the rest of the band before you perform an exercise. If you are using a doorknob or piece of furniture as an anchor point, be sure that no one will open the door and that the band is firmly fixed.

## Stability Balls

A stability ball—also known as a balance ball, body ball, fitness ball, physioball, or Swiss ball—is an air-filled ball made of elastic soft vinyl and nylon with a diameter of about 55 to 75 centimeters (22-30 inches). It is a popular piece of equipment to use when performing exercises for the core and it can substitute for a bench when you perform other exercises such as the dumbbell bench press or seated shoulder press (see chapter 6). Examples of several stability balls are shown in figure 2.6.

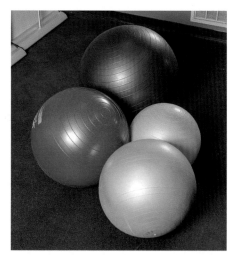

**Figure 2.6**   Various sizes of stability balls.

## Safety Considerations for Stability Balls

Be sure that the stability ball is fully inflated before using it for an exercise, especially one that requires the ball to support your body weight. It should feel very firm when you push down on it (push down on the top, not in from the side). Also, be sure to choose the right size for your height. When you sit on top of the ball with your feet flat on the floor, your thighs should be parallel to the floor.

# Weight Training Attire

Weight training requires no standardized clothing. You will see everything from tight-fitting one-piece suits (similar to those worn by wrestlers) to baggy pants and shirts. Men often wear tank tops or T-shirts and shorts. Women may wear similar clothing or choose to wear shorts over a bodysuit or shorts and a Lycra sports bra (with or without a tank top or T-shirt). Beyond your clothes, you should consider other attire while working out.

## Gloves

Weight training gloves are not a necessity, but they will help you avoid developing calluses and will provide a better grip. Buy flexible gloves with leather palms and mesh backs that fit your hands snugly.

## Shoes

Wear shoes that have firm support, especially from side to side. Look for shoes that have a normal-sized heel width, such as tennis shoes, rather than the wide or waffle heel of running shoes. Cross-training shoes are an excellent choice because they provide the best overall stability and versatility.

## Weight Belt

Another type of gear seen in weight rooms is a weight belt 4 to 6 inches (10-15 cm) wide made of leather or nylon. Weight belts add support to the lower back, especially during overhead lifting or heavy squatting exercises. See chapter 5 for more information about this popular piece of weight training equipment.

## What Not to Wear

Before you enter the weight room, take care to remove any items that may cause injury. Earrings, necklaces, bracelets, watches, and rings can catch on equipment and be ripped off or smashed, or they can create abrasions and cuts. Also, if you have long hair, secure it back so that it will not be caught in the moving parts of a machine. The same recommendation applies to oversized shirts, sweatshirts, shorts, and sweatpants.

# Weight Training Facilities

You can train in one of two places: in your home or at a fitness facility. The following section discusses the pros and cons of each option.

## Training at Home

For many people, training at home is the only practical option because of time constraints, membership cost at a fitness facility, or both. Many people simply prefer to train in their own homes. If you want to train at home, you need to consider several basic equipment and space issues.

### Room Location and Design

When selecting a place to train at home, begin by determining a suitable area for storing equipment as well as working out. The location should be out of the way of the main travel routes in your home. It should be well ventilated and well lit, and it needs at least one electrical outlet. It should also be securable if you have young children or pets. An electrical outlet offers the opportunity to plug in an mp3 player, radio, or maybe a treadmill or stair-stepping machine. If you have a choice, select an area that has a high ceiling.

The floor of a home facility is commonly carpet-covered concrete. Such a surface is better than tile or uncovered concrete because both can be slippery and easily damaged from dropping barbells and dumbbells or moving equipment. Also, arrange the tallest pieces of equipment next to the walls, but allow at least a 6-inch (15 cm) space. If you have more than one machine or bench, give yourself at least 18 inches (46 cm) between them for easy access.

### Basic Equipment Requirements

The minimum amount and type of equipment you need to use when following a basic weight program consists of a standard barbell with collars and locks, a set of adjustable dumbbells, 80 pounds (36 kg) of standard weight plates, and a bench with upright racks long enough so that you can lie down with both your head and buttocks squarely on the pad. If you are well trained—or plan to be in the future—you may need to buy an additional 135 pounds (61 kg) of standard weight plates. If the cost of equipment is a concern, resistance band training is also an option.

For more serious lifters, basic equipment needs include an Olympic bar and locks, a set of dumbbells (in 5-pound increments, possibly up to 50 pounds or more), 255 pounds (or about 120 kg) of Olympic weight plates, and a bench with upright racks to hold an Olympic bar. You may also want to buy a squat rack so that you do not have to pick up the barbell from the floor to do squats or standing shoulder presses. To hold all the weight plates, consider buying a weight tree so that the plates are not in piles on the floor.

## Training at a Fitness Facility

Selecting a fitness facility that will meet your needs is a challenge. If you need the expertise of a qualified personal trainer to help you get started, that should be the first priority when selecting where you will work out. Ideally, the facility you choose will have both qualified personnel and a variety of equipment and programs to meet your training needs.

### Training With a Personal Trainer

A well-qualified personal trainer who understands how to motivate you can make every training day an enjoyable and rewarding experience. A truly qualified personal trainer has a college degree in exercise science (or a similar area) and has earned one or more certifications in personal training, health, or fitness from a respected professional organization.

Obtain a referral from people you trust—or at least observe the personal trainer in action before making a decision. How well a personal trainer is able to make technical information understandable is essential to your success. A good personal trainer will help you understand what you are doing and why you are doing it. In addition, it never hurts to work with someone who has a motivating personality that will energize you to stick to your training program.

### Training Without a Personal Trainer

If you are new to weight training and decide to train on your own in a fitness facility, one of your first decisions concerns whether to use weight machines or free weights. Although free weights offer you the tremendous versatility of choosing among many possible exercises, they require more skill. Although machines are not foolproof, they are generally easier and safer once you learn how to use them properly. Take special care when selecting loads because sometimes even the lightest weight plate on the machine or bar may exceed your strength in a particular exercise. Also, keep in mind that the dimensions of some machines may not accommodate your physique, especially if you are short, tall, or very heavy. For those reasons, it is wise to receive instruction from a qualified professional for at least the first couple of sessions because he or she can teach you how to perform the exercise and how to make necessary machine adjustments. If you decide to use free weights, obtaining professional instruction is even more important.

# 3

# Success Starts Here

This chapter takes you through the steps in determining your fitness level, selecting a training goal, and establishing training loads. It also covers safety guidelines and training tips.

After you decide to begin a weight training program, it is natural to do too much too soon. If you are out of shape, remember that you did not get that way in a couple of days. You cannot get back into shape in a couple of days, either, so don't try! Your attempts to do so might lead to excessive muscle soreness, extreme fatigue, reduced enthusiasm about resuming training, and injury. Also, use the assessment for physical readiness to determine whether

---

### Assessing Your Physical Readiness

If you answer yes to any of the following questions, you should talk with your doctor *before* beginning a weight training program.

| Yes | No | |
|-----|-----|---|
| ___ | ___ | Are you over age 55 (female) or 45 (male) and not accustomed to exercise? |
| ___ | ___ | Do you have a history of heart disease? |
| ___ | ___ | Has a doctor ever said your blood pressure was too high? |
| ___ | ___ | Are you taking any prescription medications, such as those for heart problems or high blood pressure? |
| ___ | ___ | Have you ever experienced chest pain, spells of severe dizziness, or fainting? |
| ___ | ___ | Do you have a history of respiratory problems, such as asthma? |
| ___ | ___ | Have you had surgery or had problems with your bones, muscles, tendons, or ligaments (especially in your back, shoulders, or knees) that might be aggravated by an exercise program? |
| ___ | ___ | Is there a good physical or health reason not already mentioned here that you should not follow a weight training program? |

---

you need to make an appointment with your doctor before you start your weight training program.

# Test Your Weight Training Fitness

Knowing your fitness status will enable you to select a training level that matches your current abilities and will help you establish reasonable goals. Determine your current fitness level for weight training by using the bench press test. The results of this test will give you a general idea of your readiness to begin weight training. Refer to chapter 6 for photos and an explanation of how to perform the free-weight bench press exercise.

## BENCH PRESS TEST

### Equipment
- A 35-pound (or 15 kg) barbell for women or an 80-pound (35 kg) barbell for men
- Flat bench press bench (with upright racks to hold the bar)

### Directions
1. Seek the help of a qualified person to spot (supervise) you as you perform the test.
2. Lie on your back with your head, shoulders, upper back, and buttocks on the bench and your legs straddled with feet flat on the floor.
3. With your palms facing up, grip the bar at a position slightly wider than shoulder width.
4. With the spotter's assistance, move the bar upward and away from the uprights until your elbows are fully extended and the bar is directly over the middle of your chest.
5. Lower the bar to touch your chest lightly and briefly.
6. Push the bar upward until your elbows are fully extended (but not force-fully locked out); this action completes the first repetition.
7. Continue lowering and pressing the barbell until you cannot complete another repetition with proper technique. Do not pause to rest between repetitions. If you do, the test is over.
8. Record the number of repetitions that you complete.

### Important!

Perform each repetition in a slow, controlled manner. Allow one to two seconds to push the bar to the extended-elbow position and one to two seconds to perform the downward movement to the chest. Each repetition should take two to four seconds to complete. Do not bounce the bar off your chest. Remember to exhale when pushing upward and inhale as you lower the bar, especially when the repetitions become more difficult to complete.

To determine your rating, refer to the top half of table 3.1 if you are male and the lower half if you are female. Find your age in the ranges and follow down the column to one of the three rows of repetition ranges that includes the number that you completed. Then move over to the far-left column to determine the status of your weight training fitness.

Table 3.1  Muscular Fitness Norms of the Bench Press Test*

| Age | 18-25 | 26-35 | 36-45 | 46-55 | 56-65 | >66 |
|---|---|---|---|---|---|---|
| Men | | | | | | |
| Low | <20 | <17 | <14 | <9 | <5 | <4 |
| Average | 21-32 | 18-28 | 15-24 | 10-19 | 6-13 | 5-9 |
| High | >33 | >29 | >25 | >20 | >14 | >10 |
| Women | | | | | | |
| Low | <16 | <14 | <12 | <7 | <5 | <3 |
| Average | 17-27 | 15-27 | 13-23 | 8-17 | 6-13 | 4-9 |
| High | >28 | >28 | >24 | >18 | >14 | >10 |

* Weight training fitness status based on the number of completed repetitions.

Data from L.A. Golding (ed.), 2000, YMCA fitness testing and assessment manual, 4th ed. (Champaign, IL: Human Kinetics), 200-223.

Now that you have determined your fitness status, you are probably eager to begin training. But before you do, carefully read the rest of this chapter. It contains essential information on setting up a weight training program that will enable you to maximize every minute of training in a safe manner.

## Choose Your Training Goal

Focusing on a specific goal encourages you to make a commitment to training, which in turn motivates you to work out harder and more consistently. To set an effective goal, you need to take a few minutes to consider how you want your body to change because of your weight training program. Here are some questions to help you choose the right training goal:

• Are you seeking to tone and define your muscles without increasing their size significantly? If so, then the *muscle toning* workouts are probably best for you. This type of weight training program creates firmer muscles without significantly increasing their size. In addition, you will likely notice that your muscles will have better endurance; that is, you will be able to keep them active for longer periods before becoming tired.

•   Do you want to firm your muscles and increase muscle definition as well as increase size? If losing fat from certain areas while increasing the size of some muscles is your goal, then the *body shaping* workouts are the ones to choose. Body shaping programs result in many of the same changes produced by muscle toning programs, but they also can make the trained muscle larger (primarily in men). Women's bodies usually do not respond in the same way, although in some women the shoulders, thighs, arms, or back become a bit more muscular. Commonly, though, this type of weight training program will be effective at sculpting or reproportioning the body in a pleasing way.

•   Do you seek increased strength for occupational, recreational, or every-day tasks or competitive sport activities? If so, follow the *strength training* workouts. This type of weight training program focuses on making the trained muscles stronger so that they will be able to exert more force. Because this program requires the lifting of heavier loads, you should follow this program only if you are currently weight training.

## Determine Your First Workout Zone

The goal you selected identifies the type of training outcome you want. Now, you need to determine which workout zone matches your current weight training fitness status based on your score on the bench press test.

The workouts in chapters 7 to 12 are organized into six training zones based on their level of difficulty, and each zone has a specific color. The first training zone is Green and includes the easiest workouts and those that take the least amount of time to complete. The next training zone is Blue, followed by Purple, Yellow, Orange, and then Red, which contains the most strenuous workouts and requires the most time to complete.

Using table 3.2, consider both your past weight training experience (be honest!) and the result of the bench press test to select the appropriate workout zone. For example, if you are untrained (new to weight training or have done some weight training in the past but not recently) or if your bench press test revealed that you have a low fitness status, start with the Green Zone workouts. If you are trained (or you have been weight training recently) but have a low fitness status, start with the Blue Zone workouts.

Remember that the bench press test is only a guideline. If you are older than 35 or younger than 15 and have not been weight training regularly, you should start with Green or Blue Zone workouts regardless of how you scored on the bench press test. If you feel that the workouts in your starting level are too difficult, move to an easier one. A prudent approach is to be somewhat conservative, especially if you are untrained.

After you have identified your primary weight training goal and determined your fitness level for training, fill in the My Weight Training Program section.

**Table 3.2   Weight Training Fitness Levels and Recommended Initial Workout Zones**

| Weight training fitness level from the bench press test | Starting zone if you are untrained | Starting zone if you are trained |
| --- | --- | --- |
| Low | Green | Blue |
| Average | Purple | Yellow |
| High | Orange | Red |

# Follow the Secrets of Effective Training

To do all that you can to make a successful start to your new program, read the guidelines that follow and then go to chapter 4 to set up your program. Although these suggestions seem to be common sense, they can have a dramatic positive effect on how you feel while weight training.

## Train Regularly

You are virtually guaranteed success if you follow the workouts presented in this book—which means that you will be training on a regular basis. Sporadic training does not produce results! One of the most effective strategies is to work out with a partner. Being accountable to someone will make you train consistently; just find a partner who has a similar personal schedule and make plans to meet at a certain time on specific days.

## Increase Workout Intensity Gradually

To allow your muscles time to adjust to the stress of weight training, adhere to the number of training weeks listed at the top of each workout. Workouts in each training zone successively become more challenging. Following the directions will incorporate a gradual increase in the intensity or difficulty of the workouts, allowing for sufficient recovery to produce maximal results.

Do not underestimate the importance of nutrition and rest. Remember the training formula:

Regular training + balanced meals + adequate rest =
dramatic improvements

Amazingly, many people give attention to only one or two of these factors. If one is missing, the results of your program will be less than optimal. Although much has been written on the value of nutritional supplements, especially those high in protein, respected nutritionists continue to stress that balanced meals (approximately 12 percent protein, 58 percent carbohydrate, and 30 percent fat) provide dietary needs, including protein. An excellent source of nutrition information is *Nancy Clark's Sports Nutrition Guidebook, Fifth Edition* (Human Kinetics 2014).

## My Weight Training Program

1. My primary training goal is *(circle one)*
   - Muscle toning
   - Body shaping
   - Strength training
2. The result of the bench press test is _____ repetitions
3. Based on table 3.1, my weight training fitness status is *(circle one)*
   - Low
   - Average
   - High
4. Based on table 3.2, my first workout zone color is *(circle one)*

   GREEN   YELLOW

   **BLUE**   ORANGE

   **PURPLE  RED**
5. Flip ahead to chapters 7 through 12 and, based on your training goal, find your first zone workout table.

    Besides nutrition, your body needs rest to rebuild muscles after training as much as it needs training to stimulate improvement. Initially, you need to train two or three times a week. More is not always better. If you train too often, your muscles do not have enough time to receive nutrition and rebuild, and you might even injure yourself. Training smart means that you train regularly, eat balanced meals, and get enough rest.

## Develop and Maintain a Positive Attitude

Nothing worthwhile comes easily. You have to believe that weight training can produce dramatic improvements in your appearance, fitness, and physical performance—and it does. Get psyched, because you are in for a treat. Every minute of every day makes a difference. Training is uncomfortable at times, but perseverance pays off. Do not miss a training session; one missed session leads to two, two to three, and then what you could have achieved will not happen. Develop the attitude that the hour you put aside for training is the time that you are doing something for yourself. It is your time, so be selfish with it. In the end you will feel better about yourself and be healthier and more productive. Your investment in training time will yield rich rewards.

# 4

# Steps to Starting Your Program

This chapter describes two steps to follow as you prepare for your first workout. Completing these steps will enable you to start your program and prepare a workout (log) sheet for your workouts. In addition, you will find extra information about the most confusing part of a weight training program: determining the weight to use when performing each exercise.

## Step 1: Fill In Your Workout Chart

If you watch people who are in great physical condition while they work out, you will usually see them recording information on a chart, booklet, or mobile device. This practice plays an important role in your progress toward meeting your training goal because it allows you to track your improvement and stay motivated. To fill in your workout chart, follow the five guidelines in the order presented here.

### Locate Your First Workout

After determining the color zone that matches your fitness level and training experience, locate the workout in that zone that is associated with your goal of muscle toning, body shaping, or strength training. You already completed this step; go back to chapter 3 where you noted the color zone for your first workout. Note that some workouts are for a two-day-a-week program and others are for a three- or four-day-a-week program.

### Use the Workout Chart

At the top of the workout table you selected in your color zone, you will see the number of days per week that you will weight train. Find the corresponding workout chart in appendix A according to whether you will train two, three, or four days each week.

Use the workout chart that matches the number of days listed for your workout zone. Each chart covers a one-week period of training, and each workout zone covers a six-week period. Use one chart for each week that you train in a workout zone.

## Choose and Schedule Your Training Days

You should not weight train the same muscles on two consecutive days or allow more than three days to go by between workouts; doing so will compromise your improvements. So, for example, a two-day-per-week program might follow a Monday–Thursday, Tuesday–Friday, or Wednesday–Saturday (or Sunday) schedule. A program that involves three nonconsecutive training sessions could be scheduled on Mondays, Wednesdays, and Fridays or on Tuesdays, Thursdays, and Saturdays (or Sundays).

If you will work out four days a week, choose one of the three options shown in table 4.1. Choose an option that you can consistently stick with and one that is convenient for you. Each option provides two workouts each for your upper body and lower body and spreads out the workouts so that you have enough rest days between sessions that train the same muscle groups.

**Table 4.1   Options for a Four-Day-Per-Week Weight Training Schedule**

|  | Upper-body workouts | Lower-body workouts |
| --- | --- | --- |
| **Option 1** | Mondays and Thursdays | Tuesdays and Fridays |
| **Option 2** | Sundays (or Saturdays) and Wednesdays | Mondays and Thursdays |
| **Option 3** | Tuesdays and Fridays | Wednesdays and Saturdays (or Sundays) |

## Select and Record Your Exercises

Now you are ready to choose your exercises and note their names in your workout chart. If you are using an e-reader, a printable chart is also available online at www.humankinetics.com/products/all-products/Fitness-Weight-Training-3rd-Edition. Each zone workout table in chapters 7 to 12 has three columns of exercises depicting three types of exercises based on the needed equipment (or none at all!): *barbell*, *machine*, and *alternative* (e.g., body weight, dumbbell, stability ball, resistance band, or kettlebell). If you are inexperienced, you should begin with machine exercises. Barbell exercises and various alternative exercises (such as some exercises that use dumbbells or kettlebells) require more skill than machine exercises and sometimes require a spotter. Refer to chapter 6 for descriptions and photos of the exercises. The exercises listed in the exercise finder in chapter 6 denoted with an asterisk (*) are foundational exercises, especially for the Green Zone. If you are not sure what exercises to select for your program, choose one of these exercises for each muscle group because you can follow the Green Zone load guidelines in step 2 in this chapter to easily determine the loads you should use in your program.

In each zone workout table, notice that to the left of the three columns of exercises is a column that identifies the muscle group that is trained by those exercises. Based on the equipment that is available and how familiar you are with the exercises, **choose one exercise—from the three that are provided—for each muscle group**. The purpose of the three columns of exercises is to give you options based on the available equipment and your experience. Again, choose just one exercise for each muscle group and then note their names in the "Exercises" column of your workout chart. (Again, if you are reading this on an e-reader, you can download a printable chart at www.humankinetics .com/products/all-products/Fitness-Weight-Training-3rd-Edition.)

## Record Sets and Repetitions

Refer to the set and repetition information included in the selected zone workout table and transfer those numbers to your workout chart in the "Sets/reps" column. Be sure to record the correct set and repetition information for each exercise; for some workouts, the recommendations vary across the exercises.

Your workout chart provides a diary of each training session. Fill in all of the information as you go along to monitor your progress as you work out on a regular basis.

# Step 2: Determine Training Loads

Determining the load, or weight, that you can lift for the recommended number of repetitions for each exercise is a challenge. This step provides a description of two methods to help you accomplish this task. If you are new to weight training and have no experience in selecting training loads, use the Green Zone load guidelines. If you are experienced, use the Blue-Red Zone load guidelines.

## Green Zone Load Guidelines

Tables 4.2 (for women) and 4.3 (for men) are load calculation tables that will help you determine the right training loads for the Green Zone workouts. The exercises included in those tables are the same exercises that are asterisked in the exercise finder in chapter 6. The following sections describe the process for calculating, testing, and adjusting a load to determine the weight for each exercise that you will use for your first workout.

### Calculate the Trial Load

The first step is to determine an initial load for each exercise based on the exercise and your sex:

1. Look at the names of the exercises you recorded on your workout chart and then highlight the corresponding *factor* (a number that represents a certain percentage of your body weight) on table 4.2 or 4.3. Notice that men and women use different factors as seen in the two tables.

## Table 4.2   Load Calculations for Women

| Exercise | BW | Factor | Trial load* | Repetitions completed | Adj. | Training load* |
|---|---|---|---|---|---|---|
| **Chest** | | | | | | |
| Bench press | ____ | × 0.35 = | ____ | ____ | ____ | ____ |
| Pec deck | ____ | × 0.27 = | ____ | ____ | ____ | ____ |
| Chest press | ____ | × 0.27 = | ____ | ____ | ____ | ____ |
| **Back** | | | | | | |
| Bent-over row | ____ | × 0.35 = | ____ | ____ | ____ | ____ |
| Pullover | ____ | × 0.20 = | ____ | ____ | ____ | ____ |
| Seated row | ____ | × 0.20 = | ____ | ____ | ____ | ____ |
| Low-pulley row | ____ | × 0.25 = | ____ | ____ | ____ | ____ |
| **Shoulders** | | | | | | |
| Standing press | ____ | × 0.22 = | ____ | ____ | ____ | ____ |
| Shoulder press | ____ | × 0.20 = | ____ | ____ | ____ | ____ |
| **Biceps** | | | | | | |
| Biceps curl | ____ | × 0.23 = | ____ | ____ | ____ | ____ |
| Low-pulley curl | ____ | × 0.15 = | ____ | ____ | ____ | ____ |
| Preacher curl | ____ | × 0.12 = | ____ | ____ | ____ | ____ |
| **Triceps** | | | | | | |
| Lying triceps extension | ____ | × 0.12 = | ____ | ____ | ____ | ____ |
| Triceps extension | ____ | × 0.13 = | ____ | ____ | ____ | ____ |
| Triceps pushdown | ____ | × 0.19 = | ____ | ____ | ____ | ____ |
| **Legs** | | | | | | |
| Leg press | ____ | × 1.0 = | ____ | ____ | ____ | ____ |
| Lunge (DB) | 5 pounds (~2.5 kg) each hand | | | | | |
| **Core** | | | | | | |
| Abdominal crunch | ____ | × 0.20 = | ____ | ____ | ____ | ____ |

From *Fitness Weight Training, 3rd edition* by Thomas R. Baechle and Roger W. Earle, 2014, Champaign, IL: Human Kinetics.

The calculated trial load is designed to allow 12 to 15 repetitions. BW = body weight. DB = dumbbells. Remember to use a maximum body weight of 140 pounds (64 kg) for women. Consult chapter 6 for descriptions of proper exercise technique.

* Round down the nearest 5-pound (or 2.5 kg if you are using plates in kilograms) increment, or if you chose a machine exercise, select the closest (lighter) weight stack plate.

2. Record your body weight in the blank in the column labeled "BW" next to the "Factor" column. *Important:* Men weighing 175 pounds (79 kg) or more and women weighing 140 pounds (64 kg) or more should record 175 (79 kg) and 140 (64 kg), respectively, for their body weight in the "BW" column—*not* their actual body weight.

## Table 4.3  Load Calculations for Men

| Exercise | BW | Factor | Trial load* | Repetitions completed | Adj. | Training load* |
|---|---|---|---|---|---|---|
| **Chest** | | | | | | |
| Bench press | ____ | × 0.60 = | ____ | ____ | ____ | ____ |
| Pec deck | ____ | × 0.55 = | ____ | ____ | ____ | ____ |
| Chest press | ____ | × 0.55 = | ____ | ____ | ____ | ____ |
| **Back** | | | | | | |
| Bent-over row | ____ | × 0.45 = | ____ | ____ | ____ | ____ |
| Pullover | ____ | × 0.40 = | ____ | ____ | ____ | ____ |
| Seated row | ____ | × 0.40 = | ____ | ____ | ____ | ____ |
| Low-pulley row | ____ | × 0.45 = | ____ | ____ | ____ | ____ |
| **Shoulders** | | | | | | |
| Standing press | ____ | × 0.38 = | ____ | ____ | ____ | ____ |
| Shoulder press | ____ | × 0.35 = | ____ | ____ | ____ | ____ |
| **Biceps** | | | | | | |
| Biceps curl | ____ | × 0.30 = | ____ | ____ | ____ | ____ |
| Low-pulley curl | ____ | × 0.25 = | ____ | ____ | ____ | ____ |
| Preacher curl | ____ | × 0.20 = | ____ | ____ | ____ | ____ |
| **Triceps** | | | | | | |
| Lying triceps extension | ____ | × 0.21 = | ____ | ____ | ____ | ____ |
| Triceps extension | ____ | × 0.35 = | ____ | ____ | ____ | ____ |
| Triceps pushdown | ____ | × 0.32 = | ____ | ____ | ____ | ____ |
| **Legs** | | | | | | |
| Leg press | ____ | × 1.3 = | ____ | ____ | ____ | ____ |
| Lunge (DB) | 10 pounds (~5 kg) each hand | | | | | |
| **Core** | | | | | | |
| Abdominal crunch | ____ | × 0.20 = | ____ | ____ | ____ | ____ |

From *Fitness Weight Training, 3rd edition* by Thomas R. Baechle and Roger W. Earle, 2014, Champaign, IL: Human Kinetics.

The calculated trial load is designed to allow 12 to 15 repetitions. BW = body weight. DB = dumbbells. Remember to use a maximum body weight of 175 pounds (79 kg) for men. Consult chapter 6 for descriptions of proper exercise technique.

* Round down the nearest 5-pound (or 2.5. kg if you are using plates in kilograms) increment, or if you chose a machine exercise, select the closest (lighter) weight stack plate.

3. To determine the trial load, multiply your body weight by the factor. The load is called a *trial load* because you are trying it out to see whether it will result in the required number of repetitions.

4. Round off the trial load to the nearest 5-pound (or 2.5 kg if you are using plates in kilograms) increment (by rounding down), or if you choose a machine exercise, select the closest weight stack plate (again, by rounding down).

Table 4.4 shows an example of how to use table 4.2 to establish a trial load. In this example, the factor associated with the bench press exercise is 0.35 (for women). If the woman weighs 120 pounds (55 kg), the trial load is 40 pounds (18 kg) after rounding it down from 42 pounds (19 kg).

### Table 4.4 Example of Calculating the Trial Load

| Exercise | BW | Factor | Trial load | Repetitions completed | Adj. | Training load |
|---|---|---|---|---|---|---|
| **Chest** | | | | | | |
| Bench press | 120 | × 0.35 = | 40* | ___ | ___ | ___ |
| Pec deck | ___ | × 0.27 = | ___ | ___ | ___ | ___ |
| Chest press | ___ | × 0.27 = | ___ | ___ | ___ | ___ |

* Rounded down from 42 pounds.

## Try Out the Trial Load

After warming up, perform as many repetitions as you can—using proper technique—with the trial load, and record that number in the "Repetitions completed" column in table 4.2 or 4.3. (You can also go to www.humankinetics .com/products/all-products/Fitness-Weight-Training-3rd-Edition to download tables 4.2 and 4.3.) Do not be concerned if the trial load is too light or too heavy to use as the actual load for your first workout; the next step explains how to make adjustments. Note, though, that if the weight is light enough that you can perform over 20 repetitions, you can stop at 20; there is no extra benefit to perform more than 20. Again, it is very important that you warm up—in each exercise—before trying out the trial load.

## Make Load Adjustments (Green Zone)

The factors in tables 4.2 and 4.3 are designed to result in a load that you can perform for 12 to 15 repetitions. Because of the wide range of people who use this book to create a weight training program, it is likely that the load will not be quite right—it is either too light or too heavy. Therefore, if you could perform more than 15 repetitions or could not perform at least 12 repetitions, use table 4.5 to help you adjust the trial load to yield a more desirable starting load for each exercise.

Table 4.6 is an example of how to use the load calculation and load adjustment tables to determine an appropriate workout load. In this example, a 170-pound (77 kg) man needs to calculate his workout load for the bench press. For men, the factor associated with this exercise is 0.60 (see table 4.3). Therefore, the man's trial load is 100 pounds (170 × 0.60 is 102 pounds, and then rounded down to 100), and he was able to perform 9 repetitions with this load. Because the goal was to complete 12 to 15 repetitions, the trial load was too heavy. According to the load adjustment table (table 4.5), completing 9 repetitions requires an adjustment of −10 pounds. So, in this example, the man

Table 4.5 Adjusting the Load

| Repetitions completed | Adjustment (in pounds) |
|---|---|
| <7 | −15 |
| 8-9 | −10 |
| 10-11 | −5 |
| 12-15 | 0 |
| 16-17 | +5 |
| 18-19 | +10 |
| >20 | +15 |

Reprinted, by permission, from T.R. Baechle and R.W. Earle, 2012, *Weight training: Steps to success*, 4th ed. (Champaign, IL: Human Kinetics), 37.

Table 4.6 Example of Adjusting the Load

| Exercise | BW | Factor | Trial load | Repetitions completed | Adj. | Training load |
|---|---|---|---|---|---|---|
| | | | Chest | | | |
| Bench press | 170 | × 0.60 = | 100* | 9 | −10 | 90 |
| Pec deck | ___ | × 0.55 = | ___ | ___ | ___ | ___ |
| Chest press | ___ | × 0.55 = | ___ | ___ | ___ | ___ |

* Rounded down from 102 pounds.

needs to subtract 10 pounds from the trial load to yield a workout load of 90 pounds, the number that is in the far-right "Training load" column in the load calculation table (table 4.6) for the bench press exercise.

## Blue-Red Zone Load Guidelines

If you choose one of the more advanced workout levels, you can use the *one-repetition maximum (1RM)* procedure for determining loads for some of the exercises in your workout. This method is significantly more demanding than using the Green Zone load guidelines because the 1RM procedure requires you to lift the most weight that you can in a single all-out effort. This 1RM approach is appropriate only for exercises that train larger muscles (such as the chest, shoulders, and thighs) and involve two or more joints changing angles as the exercises are performed. Exercises that meet these criteria are called *multijoint exercises* (abbreviated as MJEs); they are more intense than exercises that isolate one muscle and involve movement at only one joint (called *single-joint exercises* and abbreviated as SJEs). Attempting 1RM in SJEs that recruit smaller muscle groups (the forearms, arms, neck, and calves) increases your chances for injury because those muscles and their associated joints may not be able to withstand the stress of lifting maximal loads. **Therefore, you should not use the 1RM procedure to determine loads for SJEs**. Table 4.7 lists the MJEs in this book that you can use in the 1RM procedure to determine workout loads.

## Table 4.7   Exercises Suitable for the 1RM Procedure

| Muscle group | Multijoint exercise (MJE) | |
|---|---|---|
| Chest | *Bench press* | Chest press |
| | *Incline bench press* | *Bench press (DB)* |
| Shoulders | *Standing press* | *Shoulder press (DB)* |
| | Shoulder press | |
| Thighs | *Squat* | *Squat (DB)* |
| | Hip sled | *Step-up (DB)* |
| | Leg press | |

Free-weight versions of the boldfaced and *italicized* exercises require an experienced spotter. DB = dumbbell (*Note:* Although the dumbbell exercises listed here are MJEs, exercise caution when using the 1RM procedure; only very advanced and well-trained individuals should consider testing their strength with these exercises. Ideally, the barbell version should be selected instead.)

### 1RM Procedure for MJEs

Essentially, the 1RM procedure involves starting with a light warm-up load and progressively adding weight until, after five or six sets, the 1RM (again, the most weight you can lift for one repetition) is determined.

To be safe, you should approach the 1RM with these priorities in mind:

- Perform the exercise with proper technique.
- Select the correct load to lift in each 1RM attempt.
- Use a two- to five-minute rest period between attempts.
- Ask a qualified person to spot you (if the exercise requires it).

If you have never attempted a 1RM, be sure you try it only under the watchful eye of a qualified personal trainer. Some free-weight exercises require a skilled spotter, and all exercises require a reasonable level of previous physical training before performing the 1RM procedure. Unless you are completely confident in your ability to perform the exercise correctly or have access to a qualified professional who can teach you the proper techniques, do not attempt to perform a 1RM! Table 4.8 lists the steps in determining a 1RM for your MJEs.

### Determine Training Loads for MJEs

Testing for your 1RM is the first of two steps in determining a training load for MJEs. The second step involves the use of table 4.9 in conjunction with the zone workout you plan to follow.

Look at the table for your first workout of your color zone; the third column gives you the required number of repetitions to perform in each exercise. Now locate the "Goal repetitions" column in table 4.9 that includes (or is the closest to) the number of repetitions from your zone workout table. Next, in the left-side "1RM" column of table 4.9, find the row with the number closest to your 1RM. Where the "Goal repetitions" column and the 1RM row intersect

### Table 4.8 Assessing the 1RM for MJEs in Blue-Red Zone Workouts

| Set # | Estimate of the appropriate load (or the amount of weight to add) | Perform this number of repetitions | Rest for this long |
|---|---|---|---|
| 1 | You can perform 20 repetitions with this load, but . . . | 12 | 2 minutes |
| 2 | You can perform 10 repetitions with this load, but . . . | 6 | 2 minutes |
| 3 | You can perform 5 to 6 repetitions with this load, but . . . | 3 | 2 minutes |
| 4 | (add 10 pounds, or ~5 kg) | 1 | 3 to 5 minutes |
| 5 | (add 10 pounds, or ~5 kg) | 1 | 3 to 5 minutes |
| *6 | (add 10 pounds, or ~5 kg) | 1 | – |

*Continue adding 10 pounds (~5 kg) as needed until you can no longer lift the weight. When failure occurs, reduce the load by 5 pounds (~2.5 kg), rest three to five minutes, and try to perform one repetition. The heaviest weight you successfully lifted is your 1RM for that exercise.

is the recommended training load for the MJE. If needed, round down to the nearest 5-pound (or 2.5 kg if you are using plates in kilograms) increment, or if you chose a machine exercise, select the closest (lighter) weight stack plate.

For example, imagine that you are following the Orange Zone strength training workout 1. The goal repetitions for an MJE such as the shoulder press are listed as 6 to 8, and your 1RM for this exercise is 170. The "6 to 7 goal repetitions" column and the 170 "1RM" row intersect at the number 141. By rounding off to the nearest 5 pounds, you determine a training load of 140 for the shoulder press. You then enter this value on your workout chart.

### Table 4.9 Determining Training Loads for MJEs in the Blue-Red Zone Workouts

| 1RM | Goal repetitions | | | | | |
|---|---|---|---|---|---|---|
| | 12-15 | 10-12 | 8-9 | 6-7 | 4-5 | 2-3 |
| | Training loads (pounds)* | | | | | |
| 30 | 18 | 21 | 23 | 25 | 26 | 28 |
| 35 | 21 | 24 | 27 | 29 | 30 | 33 |
| 40 | 24 | 28 | 31 | 33 | 35 | 37 |
| 45 | 27 | 31 | 35 | 37 | 39 | 42 |
| 50 | 30 | 35 | 39 | 42 | 44 | 47 |
| 55 | 33 | 38 | 42 | 46 | 48 | 51 |
| 60 | 36 | 42 | 46 | 50 | 52 | 56 |
| 65 | 39 | 45 | 50 | 54 | 57 | 60 |
| 70 | 42 | 49 | 54 | 58 | 61 | 65 |

> continued

Table 4.9 > *continued*

| 1RM | Goal repetitions | | | | | |
|---|---|---|---|---|---|---|
| | 12-15 | 10-12 | 8-9 | 6-7 | 4-5 | 2-3 |
| | Training loads (pounds)* | | | | | |
| 75 | 45 | 52 | 58 | 62 | 65 | 70 |
| 80 | 48 | 56 | 62 | 66 | 70 | 74 |
| 85 | 51 | 59 | 65 | 71 | 74 | 79 |
| 90 | 54 | 63 | 69 | 75 | 78 | 84 |
| 95 | 57 | 66 | 73 | 79 | 83 | 88 |
| 100 | 60 | 70 | 77 | 83 | 87 | 93 |
| 110 | 66 | 77 | 85 | 91 | 96 | 102 |
| 120 | 72 | 84 | 92 | 100 | 104 | 112 |
| 130 | 78 | 91 | 100 | 108 | 113 | 121 |
| 140 | 84 | 98 | 108 | 116 | 122 | 130 |
| 150 | 90 | 105 | 116 | 125 | 131 | 140 |
| 160 | 96 | 112 | 123 | 133 | 139 | 149 |
| 170 | 102 | 119 | 131 | 141 | 148 | 158 |
| 180 | 108 | 126 | 139 | 149 | 157 | 167 |
| 190 | 114 | 133 | 146 | 158 | 165 | 177 |
| 200 | 120 | 140 | 154 | 166 | 174 | 186 |
| 210 | 126 | 147 | 162 | 174 | 183 | 195 |
| 220 | 132 | 154 | 169 | 183 | 191 | 205 |
| 230 | 138 | 161 | 177 | 191 | 200 | 214 |
| 240 | 144 | 168 | 185 | 199 | 209 | 223 |
| 250 | 150 | 175 | 193 | 208 | 218 | 233 |
| 260 | 156 | 182 | 200 | 216 | 226 | 242 |
| 270 | 162 | 189 | 208 | 224 | 235 | 251 |
| 280 | 168 | 196 | 216 | 232 | 244 | 260 |
| 300 | 180 | 210 | 231 | 249 | 261 | 279 |
| 310 | 186 | 217 | 239 | 257 | 270 | 288 |
| 320 | 192 | 224 | 246 | 266 | 278 | 298 |
| 330 | 198 | 231 | 254 | 274 | 287 | 307 |
| 340 | 204 | 238 | 262 | 282 | 296 | 316 |
| 350 | 210 | 245 | 270 | 291 | 305 | 326 |
| 360 | 216 | 252 | 277 | 299 | 313 | 335 |
| 370 | 222 | 259 | 285 | 307 | 322 | 344 |
| 380 | 228 | 266 | 293 | 315 | 331 | 353 |
| 390 | 234 | 273 | 300 | 324 | 339 | 363 |
| 400 | 240 | 280 | 308 | 332 | 348 | 372 |

* Round down to the nearest 5-pound (or 2.5 kg if you are using plates in kilograms) increment, or if you chose a machine exercise, select the closest (lighter) weight stack plate.

## Determine Training Loads for Other Exercises

For the exercises listed in your workout that do not qualify for the 1RM procedure, try to figure out a load that is heavy or light enough so that you can lift it for the number of repetitions that is associated with your training goal (see table 4.10). It may take several trial-and-error sets to arrive at a load that is appropriate for each exercise that does not qualify for the 1RM procedure.

### Table 4.10   Load Guidelines for Exercises not Qualifying for 1RM Procedure

| Training goal | Goal repetition range |
|---|---|
| Muscle toning | 12-15 |
| Body shaping | 10-12 |
| Strength training | 8-10 |

**Resistance Band Exercises**   Unlike a barbell, dumbbell, or the weight stack of a machine, the difficulty or intensity level of a resistance band does not rely on gravity. Instead, it depends on the thickness of the band and how far it is stretched. Many (but not all) band manufacturers follow a color progression of yellow (thinnest and easiest to stretch), red, green, blue, black, silver, and gold (thickest and hardest to stretch). Be aware, though, that there are other color bands such as pink, maroon, light blue, orange, and brown that have a range of thicknesses also.

Because there is not a standard weight or load of a resistance band, it is difficult to determine which one (color) to start with or progress to when you are ready to increase the difficulty of the exercise. In general, though, moving from one color band to the next adds 20 to 30 percent resistance when the band is stretched to twice its resting length.

Typically, resistance band exercises are not a part of a strength training program (unless they are used to condition your smaller muscle groups), and the repetitions performed are usually in the muscle toning or body shaping ranges as seen in table 4.10.

**Kettlebell Exercises**   Because many kettlebell exercises involve multiple muscle groups, it can be difficult to determine training loads. The weight selected depends on your level of fitness and the exercise.

Most women should start with an 8 kg (18 lb) kettlebell (if you are well trained already, try using a 12 kg [26 lb] kettlebell). Men starting to work out can begin with a 16 kg (35 lb) kettlebell, while a fit man can begin with a 24 kg (53 lb) kettlebell. Despite these guidelines, your technique needs to be excellent, and you must attempt to perform the number of repetitions associated with your training goal.

### Make Load Adjustments (Blue Through Red Zones)

After you start using your training loads in your workout, you may find that they are too heavy or too light and, therefore, do not allow you to perform the desired number of repetitions. If that occurs, complete the following steps to adjust the workout load:

1. Reconfirm the number of repetitions that you are supposed to perform as listed in your zone workout table for that exercise.
2. Go to table 4.11 and find the range of "Goal repetitions" in the left-side column that includes the number of repetitions from your zone workout table.
3. Under the heading "Repetitions completed," find the repetition range that includes the number of repetitions that you were able to complete with the workout load.
4. Where the "Goal repetitions" row and "Repetitions completed" column intersect is the load adjustment.
5. To establish a new training load for your next workout, decrease (−) or increase (+) the original load.
6. Repeat this procedure as needed; sometimes you may have to make several adjustments to determine an accurate training load.

For example, your zone training workout directs you complete 10 repetitions ("Goal repetitions") for the bench press exercise and you determine that your initial load is 110 pounds (50 kg). After a warm-up, you are able to perform 15 repetitions. As seen in table 4.11, a "Goal repetitions" of 10 (within the 10- to 11-repetition range) intersects the "Repetitions completed" of 15 (within the 14- to 15-repetition range) at +10. When you add 10 pounds to the original 110-pound load, the adjusted load is 120 pounds (55 kg).

### Table 4.11 Adjusting Loads for the Blue-Red Zone Workouts

| Goal repetitions | Repetitions completed | | | | | | | | | |
|---|---|---|---|---|---|---|---|---|---|---|
| | >18 | 16-17 | 14-15 | 12-13 | 10-11 | 8-9 | 6-7 | 4-5 | 2-3 | <2 |
| 14-15 | +10 | +5 | | −5 | −10 | −15 | −15 | −20 | −25 | −30 |
| 12-13 | +15 | +10 | +5 | | −5 | −10 | −15 | −15 | −20 | −25 |
| 10-11 | +15 | +15 | +10 | +5 | | −5 | −10 | −15 | −15 | −20 |
| 8-9 | +20 | +15 | +15 | +10 | +5 | | −5 | −10 | −15 | −15 |
| 6-7 | +25 | +20 | +15 | +15 | +10 | +5 | | −5 | −10 | −15 |
| 4-5 | +30 | +25 | +20 | +15 | +15 | +10 | +5 | | −5 | −10 |
| 2-3 | +35 | +30 | +25 | +20 | +15 | +15 | +10 | +5 | | −5 |

Load increase (+) or decrease (−)

# 5

# Weight Train the Correct Way

Weight training is more than simply finding a barbell and pumping iron. This chapter outlines some dos and don'ts that will help you train safely and get the most out of the time and effort that you devote to training. You should read this chapter and understand the basics of proper weight training technique before you actually begin doing the exercises. In addition, knowing how to prepare to work out (the warm-up) and how to relax gradually after working out (the cool-down) will go a long way toward making each session successful.

## Learn Lifting Fundamentals

Although weight training exercises number in the hundreds, several guidelines are universal: Use a good grip, a stable body position, and effective techniques when picking up and putting down barbells, dumbbells, kettlebells, and even weight plates. You must also make good decisions about the use of weight belts and breathing technique during an exercise.

### Grip the Bar, Dumbbell, or Handle

Grasping a bar of any type involves two considerations: the type of grip to use and the spacing of your hands on the bar.

Common grips are the *pronated* (or *overhand*) grip, the *supinated* (or *underhand*) grip, and the *mixed* (or *alternated*) grip (see figure 5.1). In the overhand grip, your knuckles face up and your thumbs are toward each other. In the underhand grip, your palms face up and your thumbs point away from each other. In the alternated grip, one hand is in an underhand grip and the other in an overhand grip so your thumbs point in the same direction.

All of the grips shown in figure 5.1 are *closed grips*, meaning that your fingers and thumbs are wrapped (closed) around the bar. In an *open grip*, sometimes referred to as a *false grip*, your thumbs do not wrap around the bar. The open grip can be dangerous because the bar may roll off your palms and onto your face or foot and cause severe injury. Always use a closed grip!

Several grip widths are used in weight training. In some exercises, your hands are placed about shoulder-width apart at an equal distance from the weight plates. Some exercises require a narrower grip than this, such as at hip width. Other exercises require a wider grip. Figure 5.2 shows various grip widths. When reading the descriptions of the exercises in chapter 6, be sure to note the type of grip and the proper width for each exercise. Incorrectly placed hands can create an unbalanced grip and result in serious injury.

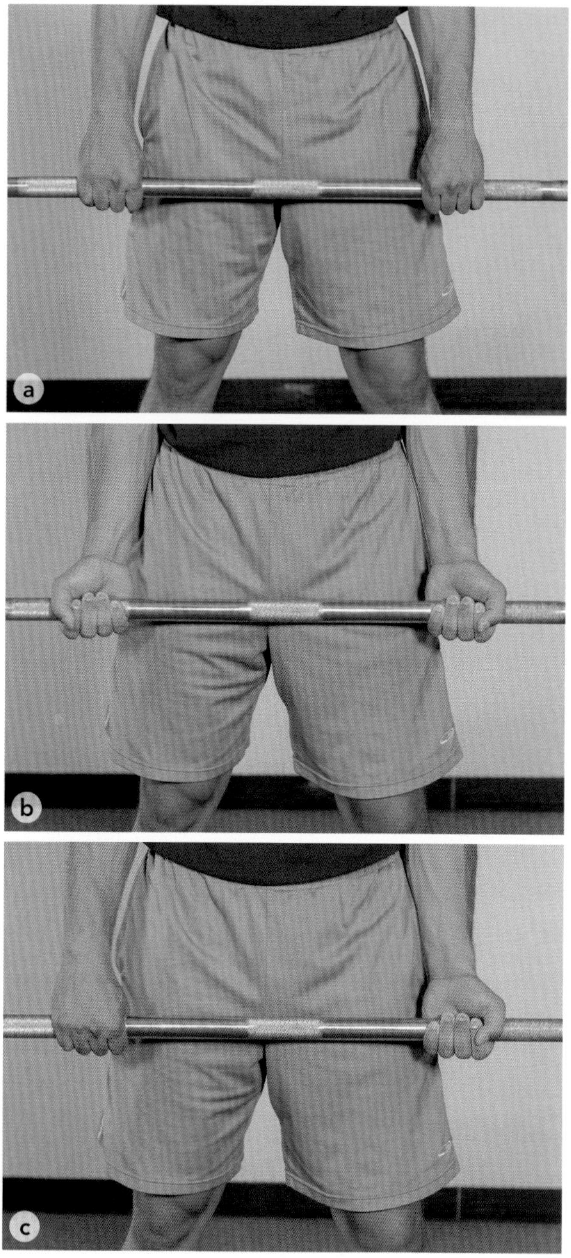

## Lift the Bar off the Floor

**Figure 5.1** Types of grip: *(a)* pronated (or overhand); *(b)* supinated (or underhand); *(c)* mixed (or alternated).

Correctly lifting the bar off the floor is important to your safety. Improper lifting can place a significant amount of stress on your neck, upper and lower back, and knees, and that stress can result in a serious injury. Establishing (or getting into) a stable body position with a balanced and secure base of support is especially important for all standing exercises—especially overhead or squatting exercises with barbells, dumbbells, or kettlebells. Furthermore, follow these guidelines to pick up a bar off the floor (or anything, for that matter):

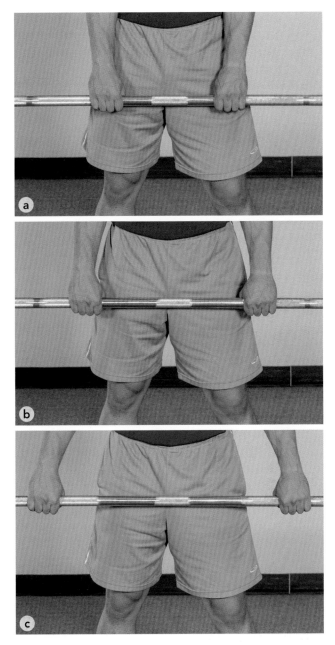

- Place your feet flat on the floor, shoulder-width apart, with your toes pointing ahead or slightly outward.

- Move the bar next to your shins (or as close as you can if there are no weight plates on it).

- Squat down by flexing both your knees and your hips (in other words, do not just bend over at your waist) and grasp the bar with a closed, overhand, shoulder-width grip.

- Position your shoulders over the bar and establish a flat

**Figure 5.2** Grip widths: *(a)* narrow width; *(b)* shoulder width; *(c)* wide width.

back (not rounded) position with your shoulders held back, chest out, head held up, and eyes looking straight ahead.

- Stand up with the bar and think, *Keep the bar close, use my legs, keep my hips low, and keep my back flat, not rounded.*

The photo sequence in figure 5.3 shows how to lift a barbell safely. Take a look at the photos before reading the next section that describes the five phases.

The preparatory lifting position (figure 5.3a) places your body in a stable position, one in which your legs—not your back—will do the lifting. Getting into the proper position is not as easy as you might think. As you squat down, one or both heels will tend to lift up, causing you to step forward to catch your balance. Remember to keep your heels on the floor! If a mirror is available, watch yourself as you squat down into the low preparatory position. Does your back stay in a flat position? Do your heels stay in contact with the floor? They should (see figure 5.3b). The most important point to remember when you lift a barbell, dumbbell, weight plate, or any object off the floor is to use your leg muscles, not your back muscles.

If you need to pull the bar to your shoulders, continue pulling it past your knees (figure 5.3c), but do not allow the bar to rest on your thighs. As you straighten your legs and hips, your hips should move forward. To pull the bar from the thighs to the shoulders effectively and safely, visualize yourself jumping up with the barbell while keeping your elbows straight (figure 5.3d), and at the very peak of the jump, shrug your shoulders and flex your elbows to catch the bar on or at your shoulders, as shown in figure 5.3e. Try to synchronize the moment when you catch the bar on or at your shoulders with the time when you land back down on the floor from the jumping portion of the exercise.

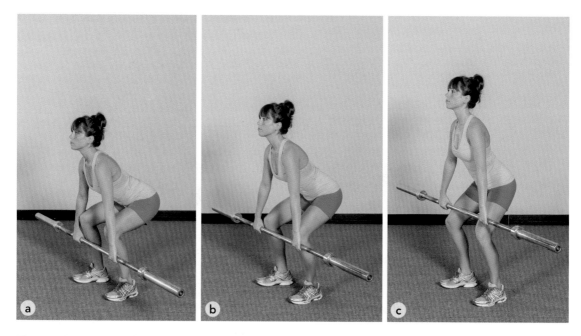

**Figure 5.3** Proper technique for lifting a barbell off the floor: (a) getting into the preparatory lifting position; (b) using your legs to lift the bar (called the first pull); (c) pulling the bar past your knees and moving your hips forward (called the scoop or transition).

## Return the Bar to the Floor

When lowering the bar or any heavy object to the floor, remember to keep the bar or weight close to you and to keep your back flat and rigid, relying on your legs to squat down to move the bar in a slow, controlled manner back to the floor. If the bar begins at shoulder height, allow the weight of the bar to pull your arms out and down, an action that will cause the bar to press against your thighs. Hold the bar briefly at midthigh before squatting down to lower the bar farther to the floor. Remember to keep your head up and your back flat throughout the return of the bar to the floor. In many ways, you will perform the movements described in figure 5.3 but in the reverse order.

## Breathe Correctly

Correct breathing while weight training can be summed up in two words: Breathe naturally. The result is an even rhythm of breathing in and breathing out without holding your breath. More specifically, you should exhale as you pass through the *sticking point*, which is the most difficult part of the work phase of the movement. For example, the sticking point of the biceps curl is approximately halfway through the upward arc of the bar; for the bench press exercise, it is where the bar is a few inches off the chest as you try to push it upward. Inhalation, then, should be during the relaxation phase as you move the bar, dumbbell, or machine back to its starting position.

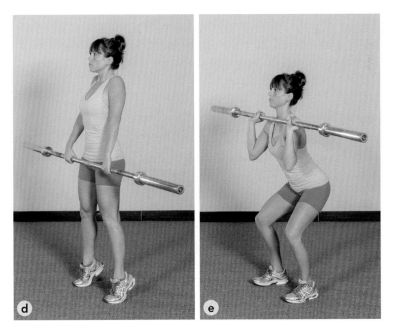

**Figure 5.3 *(continued)*** *(d)* jumping up with your elbows straight (called the second pull); *(e)* catching the bar at or on your shoulders (called the catch).

You will have a tendency to hold your breath throughout the entire exertion phase. Avoid doing this because it is dangerous! If you do not exhale, you reduce the return of blood to your heart and brain, which can make you feel dizzy and lightheaded and might cause you to faint. Holding your breath is especially dangerous when performing overhead exercises, particularly if you have high blood pressure. Put simply, proper breathing is extremely important during weight training.

## When to Wear a Weight Belt

Should you wear a weight belt? The answer varies based on the exercise and weight of the load relative to the most weight you can lift for the exercise. Here are two guidelines:

- You do not need a weight belt for exercises that do not place any stress on the lower back. Common exercises that do not require a weight belt are the lat pulldown, bench press, biceps curl, and leg extension. In other words, do not put on a weight belt for your first exercise and wear it during the rest of your workout because most exercises—when performed properly—do not apply specific stress to your lower back.
- You should definitely wear a belt when performing exercises that stress the back and involve the use of maximum or near-maximum loads. When using a belt, pull it snugly around your waist and remember that using a weight belt in and of itself will not protect you from back injuries—good technique will!

## Train With Care

The following precautions will make training safer and more effective. Often such directions or warnings are posted on a wall in a fitness facility or on a sign attached to a machine or exercise station. Although many of these precautions seem sensible, you will often see other people not following them. So be aware of your surroundings, especially during the busy times of a fitness facility before work, during the noon hour, and after work.

### Using Free Weights

Although free-weight exercises provide the greatest degree of freedom in movement, this advantage can be a liability. An increase in the options of how you can move a bar, dumbbell, kettlebell, or weight plate also means an increase in the number of potentially hazardous circumstances.

### Load Bars Properly

Take great care to load weight plates on a bar evenly and with the proper weight. If the ends of a *suspended bar* (where it is resting on the upright supports of a bench or on the hooks of a rack) are not loaded evenly, the bar may tip, possibly resulting in injury. Learning to recognize the weight of various bars and weight plates will help you in loading the bar evenly and placing the proper amount of load on the bar.

### Lock Barbells and Dumbbells

Lifting with unlocked barbells and dumbbells is dangerous. Weight plates that are not secured with locks can easily slide off the bar and land on your feet or other body parts. Before performing every set, check both locks for tightness. Do not assume that the previous person using the barbell or dumbbell tightened the locks.

### Avoid Backing Into Others

An untimely bump into another person might cause a barbell or dumbbell to fall on your head (during an overhead exercise) or face (from a lying-down exercise) or on the head or face of someone training nearby.

### Be Aware of Extended Bars

Extended bars are those that overhang or extend outward from machines (such as the lat pulldown exercise; see chapter 6), barbells supported on large racks (like on a squat rack), bench uprights, or bars held in the hands of other people who are working out. Pay special attention to bars that are positioned at or above shoulder height; serious facial injuries can result from walking into them.

### Store Equipment Properly

Each piece of equipment in the weight training area should be stored in a special location. People can trip or slip on barbells, dumbbells, and weight plates that are left unattended or not placed in their proper locations. Make sure that you put your equipment away immediately after using it, both at home and when you are working out in a fitness facility. If you have children at home, you may face an added danger if they are able to climb on equipment or try to lift plates and bars that are too heavy for them. Secure your weight training equipment so that children do not have access to it without your supervision.

## Using Machines

Although the mechanics of working out on a machine are less complicated, following a few steps will help maximize safety:

- Insert the T- or L-shaped selector key all the way in the weight stack. Also, do not use any type of key that does not come with the specific machine.

- Adjust the machine to accommodate your body size, and refer to the signs or illustrations (if provided) for the location of the adjustment knobs or dials. If there are no signs or you are not sure how to make adjustments, request help from a qualified person.
- Check that the seat, pads, and arms of the machine are locked in place so they do not slip out of position when you perform the exercise.
- Establish a stable base of support for exercises that involve placing your feet on the floor or positioning your head, torso, hips, or legs on or against the equipment.
- Fasten seat belts securely (if provided).
- Perform exercises through the full range of motion and always in a slow and controlled manner.
- Do not allow the weight plates to slam against the rest of the stack during the lowering phase or hit the pulleys during the raising phase.
- If a piece of equipment does not work properly, ask for help. Never place your hands or fingers between weight stacks to dislodge a selector key that is stuck, and keep your hands, fingers, long hair, and clothing away from moving chains, belts, pulleys, and cams.

## Warm Up and Cool Down

Preparing the body to weight train is just as important as doing the actual workout. Without a warm-up, you often will not be able to lift as much, and even attempting to weight train will not feel comfortable. After your workout, you need to decrease your activity level gradually to let your body cool down and recover.

### Warm Up

The warm-up is an essential part of any well-conceived weight training program. Warm-up activities raise the body temperature and increase blood flow to the muscles, making them more pliable and less likely to become injured when challenged to contract against heavy loads. Activities such as walking, jogging, stationary cycling, stair climbing or stair stepping, rowing, and rope skipping are excellent warm-up exercises.

Another type of warm-up involves performing the exercise that you are preparing to do but with a very light load for 8 to 15 repetitions. This specific (versus general) type of warm-up allows you to get your brain and muscles working in harmony before you tax them with heavier loads. This type of warm-up also gives you the chance to acquire a better feel for which muscles are involved and how to get them more involved in the exercise. Once you have completed 10 to 15 minutes of general warm-up, consider performing a set of 8 to 15 repetitions with a lighter load before the first actual set of an exercise.

## Stretch

You should include stretching activities for each major muscle group at the end of the warm-up and cool-down periods. Stretching is more successful after the warm-up than before it because your muscles are more flexible and more easily stretched when they are warm. Follow these guidelines as you stretch:

- Move slowly into the stretched position and stretch to a point where you can feel tension, not pain.
- Relax, inhale deeply, and then exhale.
- Hold the stretch for 15 to 30 seconds and then return slowly to the starting position.
- Perform each stretch at least twice.

The following sections describe and show the common techniques for performing basic flexibility exercises.

### CHEST AND SHOULDERS

**MAJOR MUSCLES STRETCHED: pectoralis major and deltoids**

With your elbows straight, clasp your hands together behind your back and slowly lift your arms upward. If you are not able to clasp your hands, simply reach back as far as possible. For an additional stretch, bend forward at the waist and raise your arms higher.

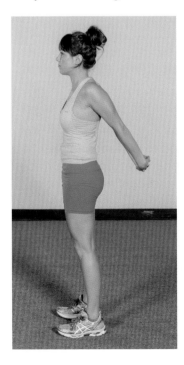

## UPPER BACK, SHOULDERS, AND BACK OF ARMS

**MAJOR MUSCLES STRETCHED: rhomboids, deltoids, and triceps brachii**

With your left hand, grasp your right elbow and pull it slowly across your chest toward your left shoulder. Repeat with your other arm.

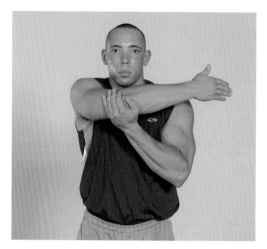

## UPPER BACK AND BACK OF ARMS

**MAJOR MUSCLES STRETCHED: latissimus dorsi and triceps brachii**

Bring both arms overhead and hold your right elbow with your left hand. Bend your right arm at the elbow and let your right hand touch your upper back. Pull with your left hand to move your right elbow slowly toward and behind your head until you feel a stretch. Repeat with your other arm.

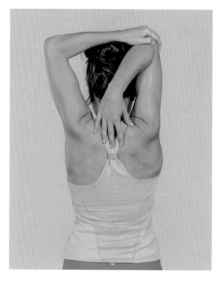

## BACK AND HIPS

**MAJOR MUSCLES STRETCHED: erector spinae and gluteus maximus**

Sit on the floor with your legs straight in front of you. Bend your right leg, cross it over your left knee, and place the sole of your right foot flat on the floor to the outside of your left knee. Next, push against the outside of your upper right thigh with your left elbow, just above your knee. Place your right hand behind you and then slowly rotate your upper body toward your right hand and arm. Repeat with your left leg placed over your right leg and rotate toward your left hand.

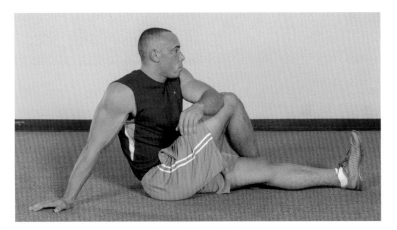

## QUADRICEPS

**MAJOR MUSCLES STRETCHED: quadriceps**

Using a wall or stationary object for balance, grasp your left foot with the left hand and pull so that your heel moves toward your left buttock (the alignment is important for avoiding stress on your knee). You should feel the stretch along the front of your left thigh. Repeat with your other leg and hand.

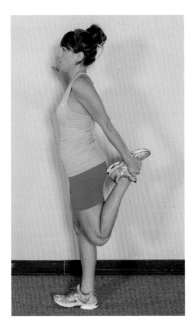

## HAMSTRINGS AND LOWER BACK

**MAJOR MUSCLES STRETCHED: hamstrings and erector spinae**

Sit on the floor with your legs straight out in front of you. Flex your right leg, rotate your right hip to point your right knee out to the side, and place the sole of your right foot lightly against the inside of your left knee. Slowly lean forward from your hips to move your torso toward your left knee. Be sure to keep the toes of your left foot pointing up with your ankles and toes relaxed. Switch the position of your legs and repeat with your right leg straight out in front of you.

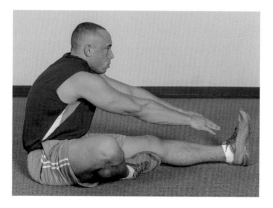

## CALVES

**MAJOR MUSCLES STRETCHED: soleus and gastrocnemius**

Stand about 3 feet (91 cm) away from a wall or stationary object. Keeping your left heel in contact with the floor, place your right foot about 1 foot (30 cm) in front of your left foot with your right knee flexed. With your left knee straight, lean forward with your entire body without flexing forward at your waist. Keep your left heel on the floor and your back straight. Repeat with your other leg.

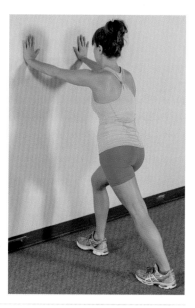

## Cool Down

Stopping abruptly when you finish your last set of exercises may cause you to become dizzy or nauseated. Cooling down with a 5- to 10-minute walk, an easy jog, or a series of stretching exercises will provide an ideal opportunity to improve your flexibility because the muscles and connective tissue surrounding the joints are warm and pliable. An additional benefit of stretching during the cool-down is that it can speed your recovery from muscle soreness.

# 6

# Weight Training Exercises

This chapter describes the most commonly accepted techniques for the exercises contained in the zone workouts. The exercises are organized into nine body areas—core, chest, back, shoulders, front of arms (biceps), back of arms (triceps), back of thigh (hamstrings), front of thigh (quadriceps), and calves—and the whole body.

Each zone workout table in chapters 7 to 12 has three columns depicting three types of exercises: *barbell*, *machine* (cam or pulley), and *alternative* (e.g., body weight [BW], dumbbell [DB], stability ball [SB], resistance band [RB], or kettlebell [KB]). The descriptions of exercise technique in this chapter also state the exercise type so you can cross-check them with the exercises in the zone workout tables.

For the exercises that also show movements, most use two photos to demonstrate proper technique. The first photo is the initial position and the second photo shows the action by way of movement arrows (if needed). In exercises for which a spotter is recommended, the spotter's role in the action is shown when possible. *Note:* Read how to identify exercises that need a spotter in the exercise description for the bench press.

The exercises denoted with an asterisk (*) in the following exercise finder are found in tables 4.2 and 4.3 and are *foundational exercises* for many of the zone workouts of this book, especially the Green Zone. If you are not sure what exercises to select for your program, choose one of these exercises for each muscle group because you can follow the step-by-step guidelines in chapter 4 to easily determine the loads you should use in your program. The page numbers listed after each exercise refer to the print book.

*Note:* There are not three exercise types for all of your body areas.

# Exercise Finder

## Core

*Barbell*

| | |
|---|---|
| Good morning | **50** |

*Machine*

| | |
|---|---|
| Abdominal crunch* | **51** |
| Back extension | **52** |

*Alternative*

| | |
|---|---|
| Back extension (SB) | **53** |
| Extended abdominal crunch (SB) | **54** |
| Side plank (BW) | **55** |
| Sit-up (BW) | **56** |
| Twisting trunk curl (BW) | **57** |

## Chest

*Barbell*

| | |
|---|---|
| Bench press* | **58** |
| Incline bench press | **60** |

*Machine*

| | |
|---|---|
| Chest press* | **62** |
| Pec deck* | **63** |

*Alternative*

| | |
|---|---|
| Bench press (DB) | **64** |
| Chest fly (DB) | **66** |
| Chest press (RB) | **68** |
| Push-up (SB) | **69** |

## Back

*Barbell*

| | |
|---|---|
| Bent-over row* | **70** |

*Machine*

| | |
|---|---|
| Lat pulldown | **71** |
| Seated row* | **72** |
| Low-pulley row* | **74** |

*Alternative*

| | |
|---|---|
| Double bent-over row (KB) | **73** |
| One-arm row (DB) | **76** |
| Seated row (RB) | **78** |

## Shoulders

*Barbell*

| | |
|---|---|
| Standing press* | **80** |
| Upright row | **82** |

*Machine*

| | |
|---|---|
| Lateral raise | **79** |
| Shoulder press* | **84** |

*Alternative*

| | |
|---|---|
| Lateral raise (RB) | **85** |
| Lateral raise (DB) | **86** |
| Shoulder press (RB) | **87** |
| Shoulder press (DB) | **88** |

## Front of Arms (Biceps)

*Barbell*

| | |
|---|---|
| Biceps curl* | **89** |
| Reverse curl | **90** |

*Machine*

| | |
|---|---|
| Low-pulley curl* | **91** |
| Preacher curl* | **92** |

*Alternative*

| | |
|---|---|
| Biceps curl (DB) | **93** |
| Biceps curl (RB) | **94** |
| Hammer curl (DB) | **95** |

## Back of Arms (Triceps)

*Barbell*
Lying triceps extension*  **96**
Seated overhead triceps
  extension  **98**

*Machine*
Triceps extension*  **100**
Triceps pushdown*  **102**

*Alternative*
One-arm triceps extension
  (RB)  **101**
Triceps kickback (DB)  **104**

## Thigh

*Barbell*
Lunge  **106**
Squat  **108**

*Machine*
Hip sled  **110**
Leg press*  **112**

*Alternative*
Front squat (KB)  **114**
Lunge (DB)*  **116**
Squat (DB)  **118**
Squat (RB)  **119**
Step-up (DB)  **120**

## Back of Thigh (Hamstrings)

*Machine*
Leg (knee) curl  **122**

*Alternative*
Leg curl (heel pull) (SB)  **124**

## Front of Thigh (Quadriceps)

*Machine*
Leg (knee) extension  **125**

*Alternative*
Wall squat (SB)  **126**

## Calves

*Machine*
Seated heel raise  **127**
Standing heel raise  **128**

*Alternative*
One-leg standing heel raise
  (DB)  **129**

## Whole Body

*Barbell*
Power clean  **130**
Push press  **132**

*Alternative*
Swing (KB)  **134**

---

*Abbreviations*
BW = body weight
DB = dumbbell
SB = stability ball
RB = resistance band
KB = kettlebell

## GOOD MORNING

**EXERCISE TYPE: barbell**

**MAJOR MUSCLES TRAINED: erector spinae, gluteus maximus, hamstrings**

### Initial Position

- Grasp the bar with a closed, pronated grip slightly wider than shoulder width.
- Position your body with the bar evenly on your upper back at the base of your neck and across the back of your shoulders.
- Slightly arch your back so that it is flat, and lift your elbows up to hold the bar in position.
- Position your feet approximately shoulder-width apart with your toes pointed slightly outward.

### Downward Movement

- Begin the exercise by slowly allowing your hips to flex. Your buttocks should move straight back during the descent.
- Maintain a flat back and high elbow position; do not round your upper back.
- Do not allow your heels to rise off the floor.
- Keep your knees slightly flexed during the descent.
- Continue the downward movement until your torso is approximately parallel to the floor.

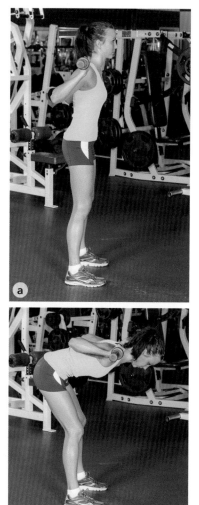

### Upward Movement

- Raise the bar by extending your hips.
- Keep your back flat and your knees slightly flexed during the ascent.
- Continue extending your hips to reach the initial position.

**EXERCISE TYPE:** machine

**MAJOR MUSCLE TRAINED:** rectus abdominis

### Initial Position

- Sit in the machine with your upper chest pressed against the pad.
- Place your feet flat on the floor under the ankle pads with your hips pressed against the small back pad.

### Forward Movement

- Lean forward to flex your torso toward your thighs.
- Do not pull the chest pad with your hands or contract your leg muscles; contract your abdominal muscles to cause the movement.

### Backward Movement

- Allow your torso to move backward to the initial position.

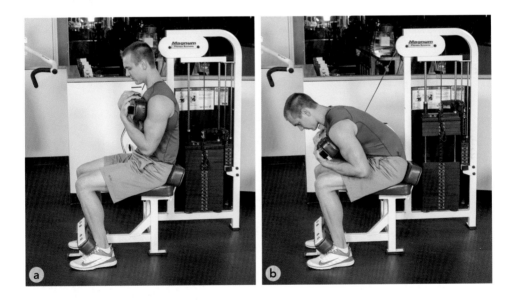

**EXERCISE TYPE:** machine

**MAJOR MUSCLE TRAINED:** erector spinae

### Initial Position

- Sit in the machine with your upper back pressed against the pad with your feet on the foot platform or under the ankle pads.
- If there are handles next to the seat, hold them with a closed, pronated grip.
- If there is a seat belt, secure it across your upper thighs just below your hips.

### Backward Movement

- Lean backward to extend your torso, but do not arch your back.
- Do not push with your legs; contract your low back muscles to cause the movement.

### Forward Movement

- Allow your torso to move forward to the initial position.

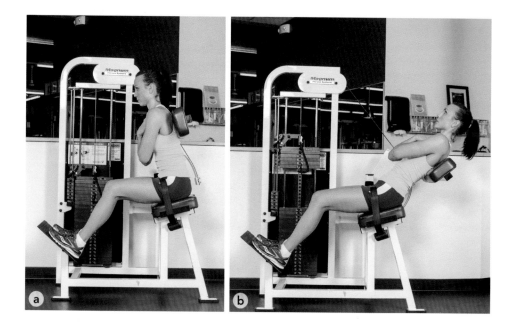

# BACK EXTENSION (SB)

**EXERCISE TYPE:** alternative

**MAJOR MUSCLE TRAINED:** erector spinae

## Initial Position

- Lie facedown on the stability ball with your navel positioned on top of the ball.
- Place your toes on the floor at least 12 inches (30 cm) apart with your knees straight (or nearly straight).
- Clasp your hands behind your head or position your hands at the sides of your head.

## Upward Movement

- Keeping your toes on the floor, lift your torso until it is straight (or moderately arched) and your chest is no longer in contact with the ball.

## Downward Movement

- Allow your torso to lower to the initial position.

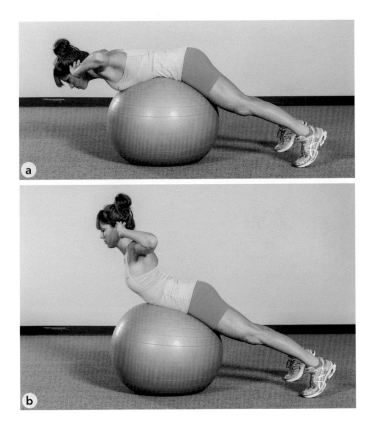

## EXTENDED ABDOMINAL CRUNCH (SB)

**EXERCISE TYPE:** alternative

**MAJOR MUSCLE TRAINED:** rectus abdominis

### Initial Position

- Lie faceup on the stability ball with the lower to middle section of your back positioned on top of the ball.
- Place your feet flat on the floor about hip-width apart with your thighs, hips, and lower abdomen approximately parallel to the floor.
- Place your hands behind or at the sides of your head or cross your arms over your chest or abdomen.

### Upward Movement

- Lean forward to flex your torso toward your thighs.
- Curl your torso to raise it off of the top of the ball.
- Keep your feet on the floor and your thighs and hips stationary.

### Downward Movement

- Allow your torso to lower to the initial position.

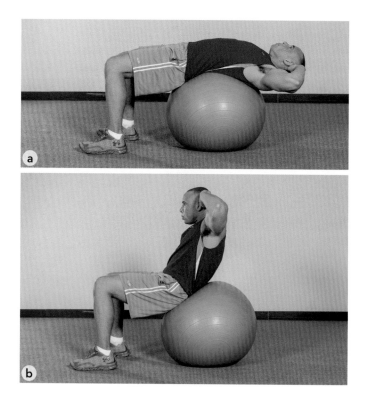

## SIDE PLANK (BW)

**EXERCISE TYPE:** alternative

**MAJOR MUSCLE TRAINED:** rectus abdominis

### Initial Position

- Lie on your right side with only your right forearm and the right side of your hips and legs touching the floor.
- Place your left hand on your left hip.
- Position your left leg on top of your right leg so they are even with each other.

### Upward Movement

- Contract your core muscles to lift your hips straight up until your whole body is in a straight line suspended off the floor.
- Keep the outside of your right foot in contact with the floor.
- Do not allow your other body segments to sag forward or backward.

### Downward Movement

- Allow your torso to lower to the initial position.
- Turn over to your left side for your next set and repeat the same movements with the outside of your left foot in contact with the floor during the exercise.

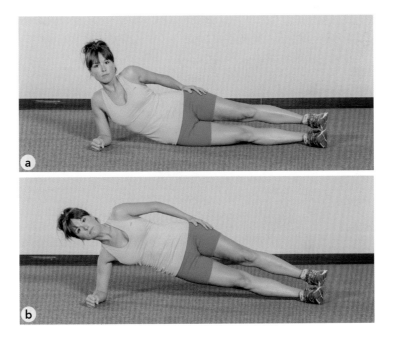

**EXERCISE TYPE:** alternative

**MAJOR MUSCLE TRAINED:** rectus abdominis

### Initial Position

- Lie faceup on the floor.
- Flex your knees to place your feet flat on the floor.
- Cross your arms over your chest or abdomen.

### Upward Movement

- Curl your torso toward your thighs until your upper back is off the floor.
- Keep your lower back and feet flat on the floor.

### Downward Movement

- Allow your torso to uncurl to the initial position.
- Do not let your hips lift off the floor.

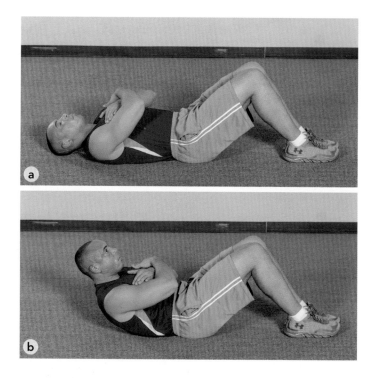

# TWISTING TRUNK CURL (BW)

**EXERCISE TYPE: alternative**

**MAJOR MUSCLE TRAINED: rectus abdominis**

### Initial Position
- Lie faceup on the floor with your feet and lower calves on a bench or chair and your knees and hips at 90-degree angles.
- Cross your arms over your chest or abdomen.

### Upward Movement
- Curl your chin to your chest and then contract your abdominal muscles to lift your shoulders off the floor.
- Immediately twist your torso so that your right shoulder or elbow points toward your left leg.
- Keep your lower back on the floor.

### Downward Movement
- Allow your torso to untwist to the initial position.
- For your next repetition, twist your torso so that your left shoulder or elbow points toward your right leg.
- Alternate the direction that you twist with each repetition.

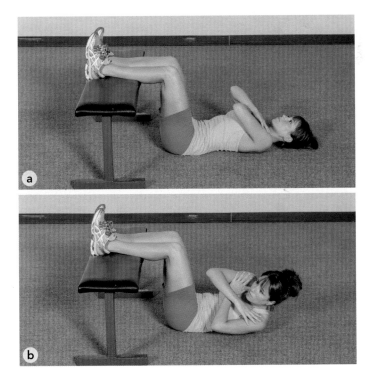

# CHEST

## BENCH PRESS*

**EXERCISE TYPE:** barbell

**MAJOR MUSCLE TRAINED:** pectoralis major

✋ **IMPORTANT:** A spotter is recommended!

### Initial Position
- Lie faceup on a bench with your head, back, and buttocks in contact with the bench and your feet flat on the floor. The bar should be over your eyes when you look at the ceiling.
- Grasp the bar with a closed, pronated grip slightly wider than shoulder width. See photo a.
- With the spotter's assistance, lift the bar off the racks and move it into a position over your chest with your elbows fully extended. See photo b.

### Downward Movement
- Allow your elbows to flex to lower the bar to touch the middle of your chest. See photo c.
- Keep a firm grip on the bar with your forearms approximately perpendicular to the floor and parallel to each other.
- Keep your head, back, and buttocks in contact with the bench and your feet flat on the floor.

### Upward Movement
- Push the bar up until your elbows are fully extended (the initial position; see photo b).
- Keep your head, back, and buttocks in contact with the bench and your feet flat on the floor.
- When you complete the set, move the bar back on the racks with the spotter's assistance.

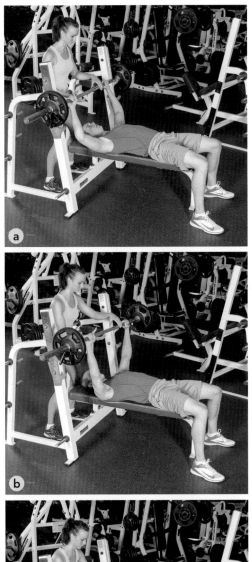

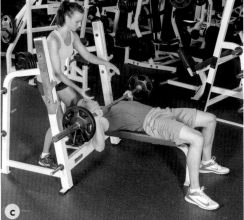

# INCLINE BENCH PRESS

**EXERCISE TYPE: barbell**

**MAJOR MUSCLE TRAINED: pectoralis major**

🖐 **IMPORTANT:** A spotter is recommended!

### Initial Position

- Lie faceup on a bench with your head, back, and buttocks in contact with the bench and your feet flat on the floor. The bar should be over and behind your head.
- Grasp the bar with a closed, pronated grip slightly wider than shoulder width.
- With the spotter's assistance, lift the bar off the racks and move it into a position over your neck and face with your elbows fully extended.

### Downward Movement

- Allow your elbows to flex to lower the bar to touch the upper part of your chest.
- Keep a firm grip on the bar with your forearms approximately perpendicular to the floor and parallel to each other.
- Keep your head, back, and buttocks in contact with the bench and your feet flat on the floor.

### Upward Movement

- Push the bar up until your elbows are fully extended (the initial position).
- Keep your head, back, and buttocks in contact with the bench and your feet flat on the floor.
- When you complete the set, move the bar back on the racks with the spotter's assistance.

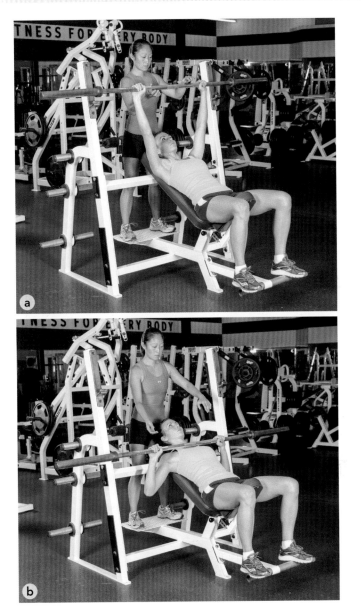

## CHEST PRESS*

**EXERCISE TYPE:** machine

**MAJOR MUSCLE TRAINED:** pectoralis major

### Initial Position

- Sit in the machine; press your head, upper back, and hips against the pads; and place your feet flat on the floor. The top of the handles should line up with the middle to upper area of your chest.
- Grasp the handles with a closed, neutral (or pronated) grip.

### Forward Movement

- Push the handles away from your body until your elbows are fully extended.
- Keep your head, back, and buttocks in contact with the pads and your feet flat on the floor.

### Backward Movement

- Allow your elbows to flex to move the handles to the initial position.
- Keep your head, back, and buttocks in contact with the pads and your feet flat on the floor.

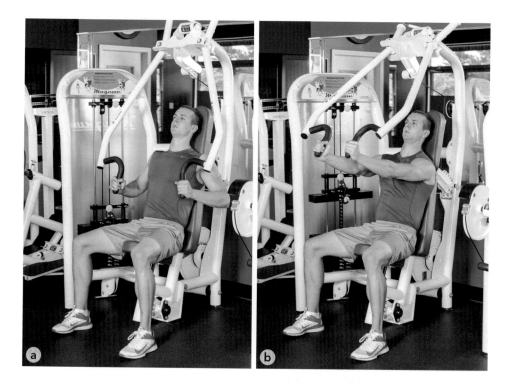

# PEC DECK*

**EXERCISE TYPE:** machine

**MAJOR MUSCLE TRAINED:** pectoralis major

### Initial Position

- Sit in the machine, press your upper back and hips against the pads, and place your feet flat on the floor.
- If the machine has arm pads, grasp the handles and press your forearms against the pads; in this position, your elbows will be flexed about 90 degrees and your upper arms should be no higher than parallel with the floor.
- If the machine only has handles, grasp them with a closed neutral grip; in this position, your elbows will be slightly flexed and your upper arms and forearms should be parallel with the floor.

### Forward Movement

- Move the handles or pads toward each other at the same rate in a wide arc.
- Continue to move the handles or pads together until they touch in front of your face. Be careful not to pinch your fingers between the handles or pads.
- Keep your feet on the floor and your upper back and hips pressed against the pads.

### Backward Movement

- Allow your arms to move out and return to the initial position.
- Keep your feet on the floor and your upper back and hips pressed against the pads.

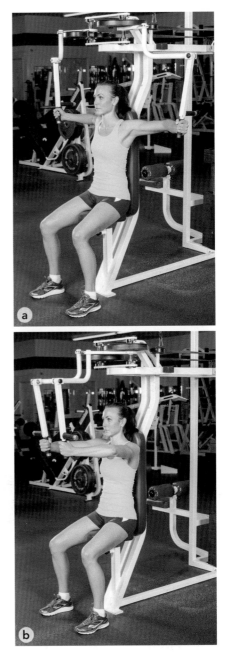

## BENCH PRESS (DB)

**EXERCISE TYPE: alternative**

**MAJOR MUSCLE TRAINED: pectoralis major**

✋ **IMPORTANT:** A spotter is recommended! The spotter assists by spotting your forearms near your wrists.

### Initial Position

- Lie faceup on a bench with your head, back, and buttocks in contact with the bench and your feet flat on the floor.
- Take the dumbbells (or have them already in your hands) from the spotter with a closed grip.
- Move the dumbbells to your chest and press them straight up until your arms are fully extended. The palms of your hands should be facing away from you.

### Downward Movement

- Allow the dumbbells to lower down and slightly out to be near your armpits and in line with the middle of your chest.
- Keep your wrists rigid and directly above your elbows with the dumbbell handles aligned with each other.
- Keep your head, back, and buttocks in contact with the bench and your feet flat on the floor.

### Upward Movement

- Push the dumbbells up and toward each other to the initial position.
- Keep your head, back, and buttocks in contact with the bench and your feet flat on the floor.
- When you complete the set, allow the spotter to take the dumbbells from your hands, or set them on the floor yourself.

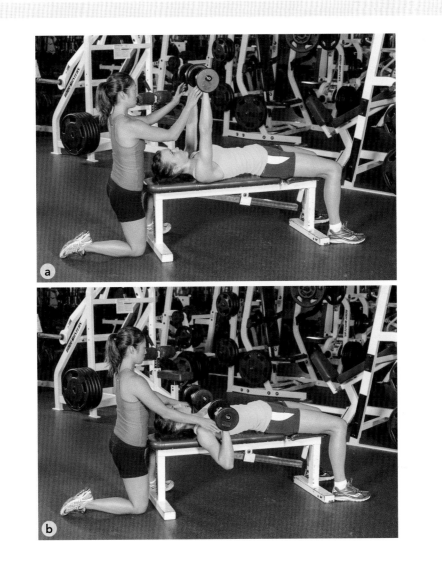

## CHEST FLY (DB)

**EXERCISE TYPE: alternative**

**MAJOR MUSCLE TRAINED: pectoralis major**

✋ **IMPORTANT:** A spotter is recommended! The spotter assists by spotting your forearms near your wrists.

*NOTE:* A spotter is not shown in the photos because it would block the view of the exercise.

### Initial Position

- Lie faceup on a bench with your head, back, and buttocks in contact with the bench and your feet flat on the floor.
- Take the dumbbells (or have them already in your hands) from the spotter with a closed grip.
- Move the dumbbells to your chest and press them straight up until your arms are fully extended.
- Rotate the dumbbells so that your palms face each other and your elbows point out to the sides.
- As you begin the exercise, slightly flex your elbows and keep them in this slightly flexed position during the exercise.

### Downward Movement

- Allow the dumbbells to lower at the same rate in a wide arc until they are level with your torso.
- Keep your palms facing each other and your elbows slightly flexed.
- Keep the dumbbells and your elbows and shoulders in one vertical plane.
- Keep your head, back, and buttocks in contact with the bench and your feet flat on the floor.

### Upward Movement

- Raise the dumbbells up and toward each other in a wide arc to the initial position.
- Keep your palms facing each other and your elbows slightly flexed.
- Keep the dumbbells and your elbows and shoulders in one vertical plane.
- Keep your head, back, and buttocks in contact with the bench and your feet flat on the floor.
- When you complete the set, allow the spotter to take the dumbbells from your hands, or set them on the floor yourself.

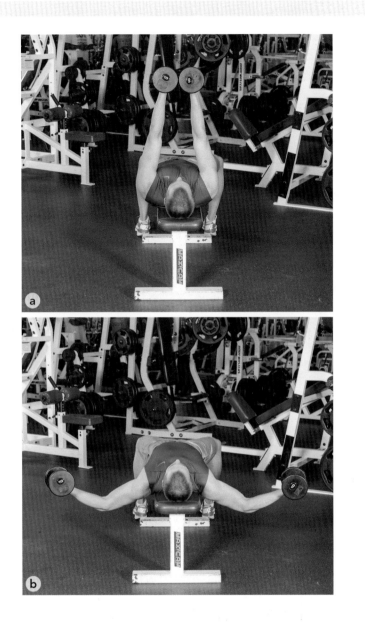

## CHEST PRESS (RB)

**EXERCISE TYPE:** alternative

**MAJOR MUSCLE TRAINED:** pectoralis major

### Initial Position

- Grasp the handles of the band with a closed, pronated (or neutral) grip.
- Evenly wrap the band around your torso at upper abdomen or midchest level.
- Stand erect with your feet shoulder-width apart and your knees slightly flexed.
- Move the handles to the sides of your torso at midchest height with your palms facing the floor.

### Forward Movement

- Push the handles away from your chest until your elbows are fully extended.
- Keep your arms approximately parallel to the floor with the rest of your body stationary.

### Backward Movement

- Allow your elbows to flex to the initial position.
- Keep your arms approximately parallel to the floor with the rest of your body stationary.

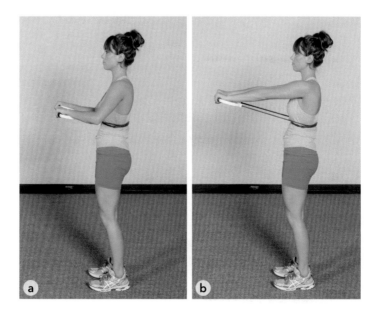

## PUSH-UP (SB)

**EXERCISE TYPE: alternative**

**MAJOR MUSCLE TRAINED: pectoralis major**

### Initial Position

- Follow the guidelines for the initial position of the stability ball back extension exercise.
- Slowly roll forward off the stability ball, place your hands on the floor, and then walk your hands forward (keeping your torso, hips, and knees rigid and in a straight line) until your shins and insteps of your feet are positioned on the top of the stability ball.
- Once in the correct body position, adjust your hands to be flat on the floor slightly wider than shoulder-width apart with your elbows fully extended.

### Downward Movement

- Allow your elbows to flex to lower your chest toward the floor while keeping your body in a straight line.

### Upward Movement

- Push with your arms to extend your elbows to the initial position.
- Do not let your hips sag or your shins and insteps to move off the top of the stability ball.

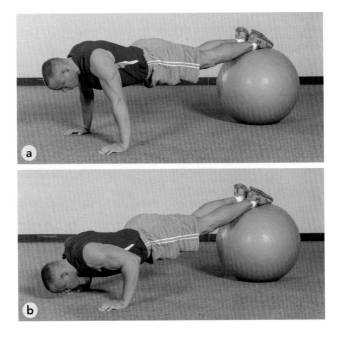

## BENT-OVER ROW*

**EXERCISE TYPE: barbell**

**MAJOR MUSCLES TRAINED: latissimus dorsi, rhomboids**

### Initial Position

- Follow the guidelines for initial position and first pull of the power clean exercise to lift the bar off the floor.
- Moderately flex your knees and flex forward to position your upper body slightly above parallel to the floor. Your upper back should be flat and rigid, not rounded or hunched over. Hold this knee and torso position during the exercise.
- Let the bar hang straight down with your elbows fully extended.

### Upward Movement

- Pull up on the bar to touch your lower chest or the upper part of your abdomen.
- Keep your wrists straight; do not curl the bar in your hands.
- Keep the rest of your body stationary.

### Downward Movement

- Allow your elbows to extend to lower the bar to the initial position.
- Keep the rest of your body stationary.
- When you complete the set, stand erect and then place the bar on the floor using a squatting movement.

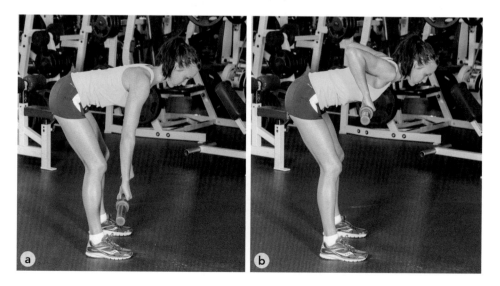

# LAT PULLDOWN

**EXERCISE TYPE:** machine (pulley)

**MAJOR MUSCLE TRAINED:** latissimus dorsi

### Initial Position

- Kneel on the floor in front (or sit in the attached seat) of a high-pulley station.
- Reach up and grasp the long bar using a closed, pronated grip wider than shoulder-width apart.
- With your elbows fully extended, lean your upper body back slightly so that you can see the bar above your face.

### Downward Movement

- Pull the bar down so that it passes close to your chin and touches the upper part of your chest.
- Keep the rest of your body stationary.

### Upward Movement

- Allow your elbows to extend to let the bar move up to the initial position.
- Keep the rest of your body stationary.

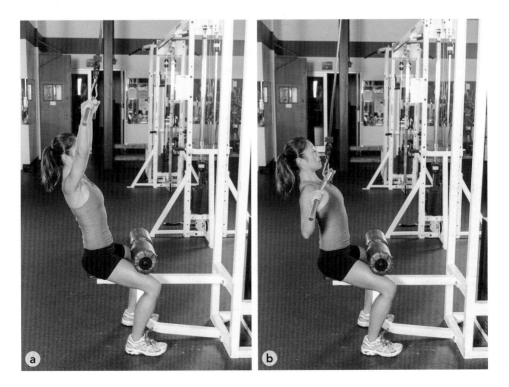

**EXERCISE TYPE: machine (cam)**

**MAJOR MUSCLES TRAINED: latissimus dorsi, rhomboids**

### Initial Position

- Sit in the machine and press your chest against the pad.
- Place your feet flat on the floor or on the foot supports (if available).
- Grasp the handles using a closed, pronated (or neutral) grip with your elbows fully extended.
- Position your upper body perpendicular to the floor.

### Backward Movement

- Pull the handles toward your lower chest or the upper part of your abdomen.
- Keep your wrists straight; do not curl the handle in your hands.
- Keep the rest of your body stationary.

### Forward Movement

- Allow your elbows to extend to the initial position.

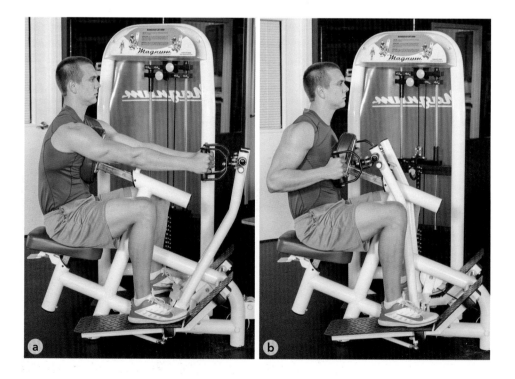

# DOUBLE BENT-OVER ROW (KB)

**EXERCISE TYPE:** alternative

**MAJOR MUSCLES TRAINED:** latissimus dorsi, rhomboids

### Initial Position

- Follow the guidelines for the initial position and first pull of the power clean exercise to lift the kettlebells off the floor.
- Flex your knees about one-quarter of the way and flex forward to position your upper body slightly above parallel to the floor. Your upper back should be flat and rigid, not rounded or hunched over. Hold this knee and torso position during the exercise.
- Let the kettlebells hang straight down with your elbows fully extended.

### Upward Movement

- Pull the kettlebells up to the sides of your torso.
- Keep your wrists straight; do not curl the handles in your hands.
- Keep the rest of your body stationary.

### Downward Movement

- Allow your elbows to extend to lower the kettlebells to the initial position.
- Keep the rest of your body stationary.
- When you complete the set, stand erect and then place the kettlebells on the floor using a squatting movement.

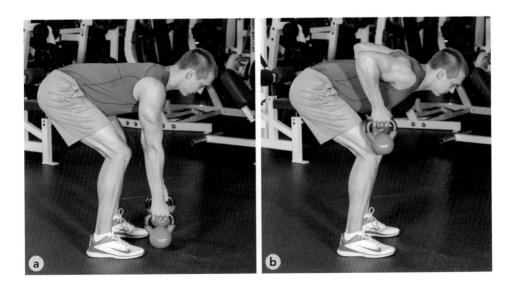

## LOW-PULLEY ROW*

**EXERCISE TYPE:** machine (pulley)

**MAJOR MUSCLES TRAINED:** latissimus dorsi, rhomboids

### Initial Position

- Sit on a long pad or on the floor (depending on the machine) and place your feet flat on the foot supports.
- Grasp the bar or handles using a closed, pronated (or neutral) grip with your elbows fully extended.
- Adjust your body to sit erect with your knees moderately flexed; hold this position during the exercise.

### Backward Movement

- Pull the bar or handles toward your abdomen.
- Keep your wrists straight; do not curl the bar in your hands.
- Keep your torso erect and your knees in the same moderately flexed position.

### Forward Movement

- Allow your elbows to extend to the initial position.
- Keep the rest of your body stationary; do not lean forward as your elbows extend.

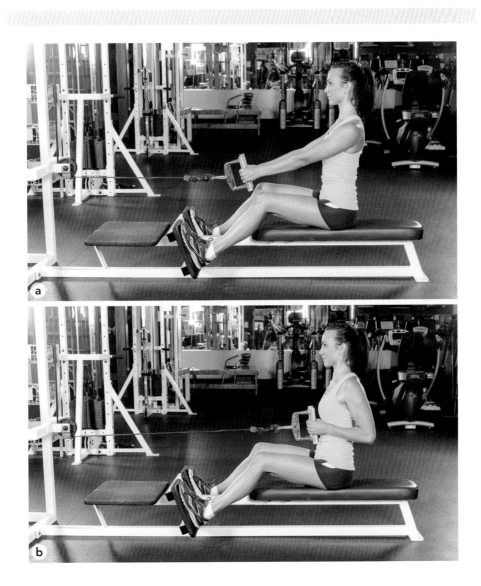

## ONE-ARM ROW (DB)

**EXERCISE TYPE: alternative**

**MAJOR MUSCLES TRAINED: latissimus dorsi, rhomboids**

### Initial Position

- Set one dumbbell on the floor on the right side of the bench.
- Stand on the right side of a flat bench and kneel on the bench with your left leg.
- Flex forward and position your left hand on the bench in front of your left knee so that your left arm and left thigh are approximately parallel to each other.
- Slightly flex your right knee and hold this position during the exercise.
- Reach down and pick up a dumbbell with your right hand using a closed, neutral grip.
- Let your right arm and dumbbell hang straight down.

### Upward Movement

- Pull up on the dumbbell to lift it to touch the right side of your torso.
- Brush the inside part of your right arm against your torso as you pull the dumbbell.
- Keep your right wrist straight; do not curl the dumbbell in your hands.
- Keep the rest of your body stationary.

### Downward Movement

- Allow your right elbow to extend to lower the dumbbell to the initial position.
- Keep the rest of your body stationary.
- When you complete the set, set the dumbbell on the floor and then stand on the left side of the bench. Repeat the movement with your left arm.

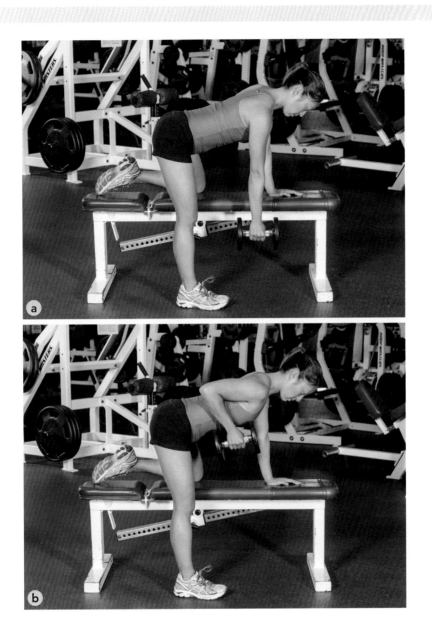

## SEATED ROW (RB)

**EXERCISE TYPE:** alternative

**MAJOR MUSCLES TRAINED: latissimus dorsi, rhomboids**

### Initial Position

- Grasp the handles of the band with a closed, pronated (or neutral) grip.
- Sit on the floor with your legs out in front of you and your knees straight.
- Evenly wrap the band around the insteps of your feet so that the band is taut when your elbows are fully extended.
- Keep your upper back flat, not rounded or hunched forward.

### Backward Movement

- Pull the handles toward the sides of your torso and ribs.
- Keep your wrists straight; do not curl the handles in your hands.
- Keep the rest of your body stationary.

### Forward Movement

- Allow your elbows to extend to the initial position.
- Keep the rest of your body stationary.

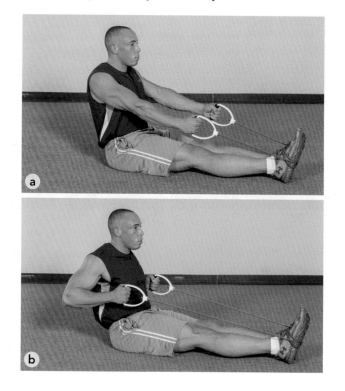

### LATERAL RAISE

**EXERCISE TYPE:** machine

**MAJOR MUSCLES TRAINED:** deltoids

#### Initial Position

- Sit in the machine, press your back against the pad, and place your feet flat on the floor.
- Grasp the handles or pads and press your upper arms against the arm pads. Your arms should be flexed approximately 90 degrees.

#### Upward Movement

- Move the handles or pads up at the same rate in a wide arc by moving only at your shoulders. Do not shrug your shoulders or pull up with your hands to help lift the weight.
- Continue to move the handles or pads up until your upper arms are approximately parallel to the floor or nearly level with your shoulders.
- Keep your feet on the floor and your back pressed against the pad.

#### Downward Movement

- Allow your arms to move down to the initial position.

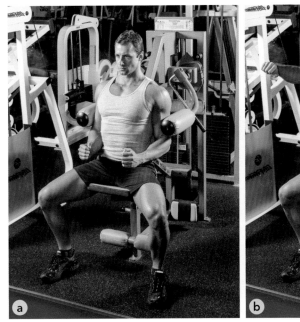
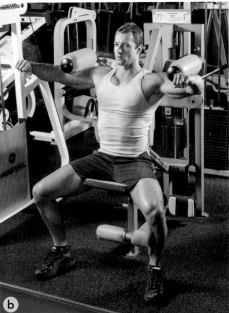

## STANDING PRESS*

**EXERCISE TYPE: barbell**

**MAJOR MUSCLES TRAINED: deltoids**

✋ **IMPORTANT:** A spotter (at least as tall as you) is recommended!

### Initial Position

*Note:* This exercise can also be performed on a seated shoulder press bench. A spotter is also recommended.

- Follow all of the guidelines for upward movement of the power clean exercise to lift the bar off the floor to your shoulders.

### Upward Movement

- As you begin the exercise, tilt your head slightly backward.
- Push the bar straight up (just missing your chin) until your elbows are fully extended.
- Keep your wrists straight and directly above your elbows.
- Do not tilt your head too far back or lean backward as you press the bar overhead.

### Downward Movement

- Allow your elbows to flex to lower the bar to the initial position.
- Tilt your head slightly so that the bar does not hit your head, nose, or chin.
- Keep your wrists straight and directly above your elbows.
- When you complete the set, place the bar on the floor using the guidelines for downward movement of the power clean exercise.

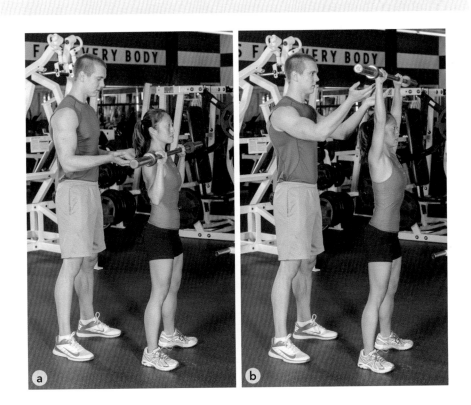

# UPRIGHT ROW

**EXERCISE TYPE: barbell**

**MAJOR MUSCLES TRAINED: deltoids, trapezius**

### Initial Position

- Grasp the bar with a closed, pronated, shoulder-width grip (or slightly narrower).
- Stand erect with your feet shoulder-width apart and knees slightly flexed.
- Rest the bar on the front of your thighs with your elbows fully extended and pointing out to the sides.

### Upward Movement

- Pull the bar up along your abdomen and chest toward your chin.
- Keep your elbows pointed out to the sides as the bar moves along your torso.
- Do not lift up your heels or swing the bar out or up; keep it under control.
- At the highest bar position, your elbows should be level with or slightly higher than your shoulders and wrists.

### Downward Movement

- Allow the bar to lower to the initial position.
- Keep your torso and knees in the same position; do not lean forward as the bar lowers.

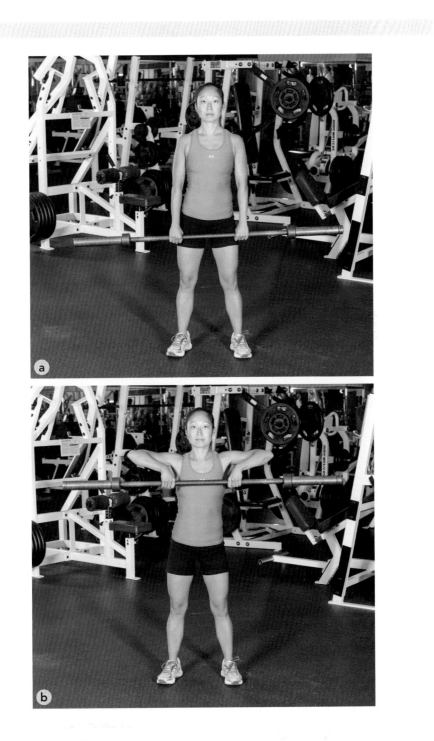

# SHOULDER PRESS*

**EXERCISE TYPE:** machine

**MAJOR MUSCLES TRAINED:** deltoids

### Initial Position

- Sit in the machine; press your head, upper back, and hips against the pads; and place your feet flat on the floor. The handles should line up with the top of your shoulders.
- Grasp the handles with a closed, pronated (or neutral) grip slightly wider than shoulder width.

### Upward Movement

- Push the handles upward until your elbows are fully extended.
- Keep your head, back, and buttocks in contact with the pads and your feet flat on the floor.

### Downward Movement

- Allow your elbows to flex to move the handles to the initial position.
- Keep your head, back, and buttocks in contact with the pads and your feet flat on the floor.

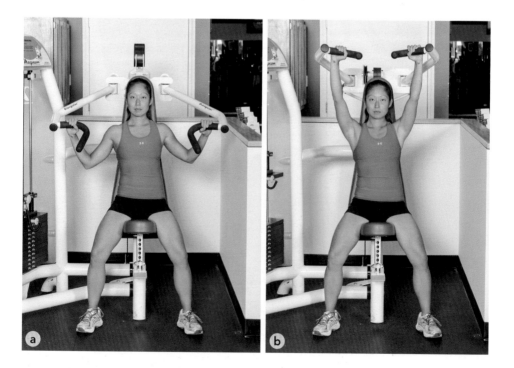

# LATERAL RAISE (RB)

**EXERCISE TYPE:** alternative

**MAJOR MUSCLES TRAINED:** deltoids

### Initial Position
- Grasp the handles of the band with a closed, neutral grip.
- Stand on top of the middle of the band with your feet shoulder-width apart or slightly narrower.
- Hold the handles out from the sides of your thighs with your palms facing inward.
- Slightly flex your elbows and hold them in this position during the exercise.

### Upward Movement
- Lift the handles up and out to the sides with your hands, forearms, elbows, and upper arms rising together. Do not shrug your shoulders to help lift the handles.
- Keep your body erect with your knees slightly flexed and feet flat on the floor.
- Continue lifting the handles until your upper arms are parallel to the floor or nearly level with your shoulders.

### Downward Movement
- Allow the handles to lower to the initial position.
- Keep your body erect with your knees slightly flexed and feet flat on the floor.

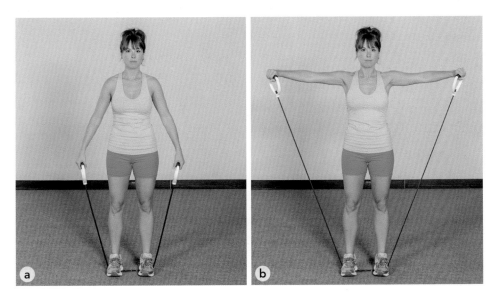

## LATERAL RAISE (DB)

**EXERCISE TYPE: alternative**

**MAJOR MUSCLES TRAINED: deltoids**

### Initial Position

- Pick up two dumbbells using a closed, neutral grip.
- Stand with your knees slightly flexed and the dumbbells positioned on the front of your thighs with your palms facing each other.
- Slightly flex your elbows and hold them in this position during the exercise.

### Upward Movement

- Lift the dumbbells up and out to the sides with your hands, forearms, elbows, and upper arms rising together. Do not shrug your shoulders or swing your arms to help lift the weight.
- Keep your body erect and feet flat on the floor.
- Continue lifting the dumbbells until your upper arms are parallel to the floor or nearly level with your shoulders.

### Downward Movement

- Allow the dumbbells to lower to the initial position.
- Keep your body erect with your feet flat on the floor.

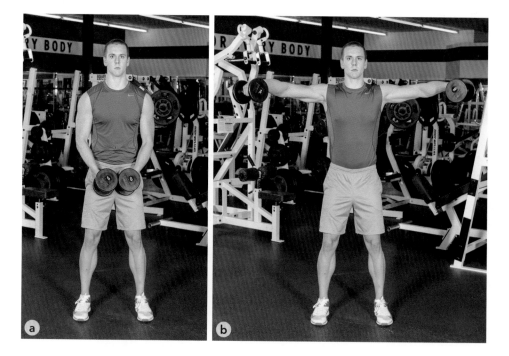

## SHOULDER PRESS (RB)

**EXERCISE TYPE:** alternative

**MAJOR MUSCLES TRAINED:** deltoids

### Initial Position
- Grasp the handles of the band with a closed, pronated grip.
- Sit erect on the floor with your legs out in front of you.
- Position your body and the band so that you are sitting on top of the middle of the band.
- Position the handles to line up with the top of your shoulders or level with your ears with your palms facing forward.

### Upward Movement
- Push the handles upward until your elbows are fully extended.
- Keep your body erect with your wrists straight and directly above your elbows.

### Downward Movement
- Allow the handles to move back down to the initial position.
- Keep your body erect with your wrists straight and directly above your elbows.

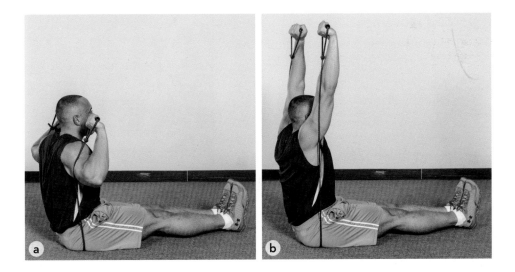

## SHOULDER PRESS (DB)

**EXERCISE TYPE:** alternative

**MAJOR MUSCLES TRAINED:** deltoids

✋ **IMPORTANT:** A spotter is recommended! The spotter assists by spotting your forearms near your wrists.

### Initial Position

- Grasp the dumbbells with a closed, pronated grip.
- Sit erect on a shoulder press bench with your head, upper back, and hips pressed against the pads. If one is not available, you can straddle a flat bench, but be sure to sit in an erect position with your feet flat on the floor.
- Move the dumbbells to position them at shoulder level with your palms facing forward. The dumbbell handles should be in line with each other and parallel to the floor.

### Upward Movement

- Push the dumbbells up until your elbows are fully extended.
- Keep your wrists straight and directly above your elbows.
- Maintain your erect torso position; do not lean back or lift off the bench as you press the dumbbells overhead.

### Downward Movement

- Allow your elbows to flex to lower the dumbbells to the initial position.
- Keep your wrists straight and directly above your elbows.
- Maintain your erect torso position.

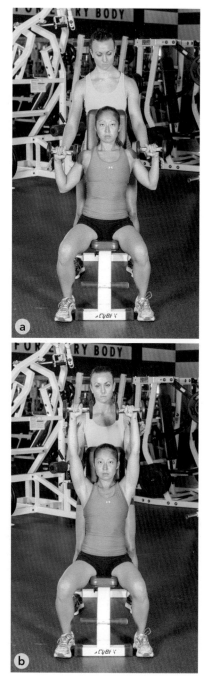

# FRONT OF ARMS (BICEPS)

## BICEPS CURL*

**EXERCISE TYPE:** barbell

**MAJOR MUSCLE TRAINED:** biceps brachii

### Initial Position
- Grasp the bar using a closed, supinated grip shoulder-width apart.
- Stand with your knees slightly flexed and the bar in front of your thighs with your elbows fully extended.

### Upward Movement
- Flex your elbows to raise the bar in an arc toward your shoulders.
- Keep your upper arms pressed against your torso during the exercise.

### Downward Movement
- Allow your elbows to extend to the initial position.
- Lower the bar in an arc until your elbows are fully extended.

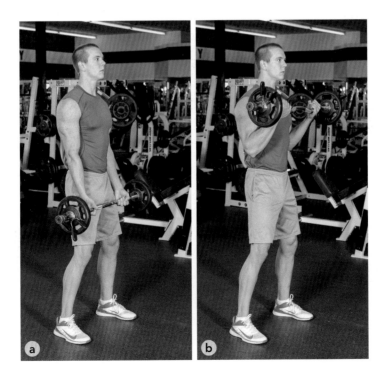

**EXERCISE TYPE:** barbell

**MAJOR MUSCLE TRAINED:** biceps brachii

### Initial Position
- Grasp the bar using a closed, pronated grip shoulder-width apart.
- Stand with your knees slightly flexed and the bar in front of your thighs with your elbows fully extended.

### Upward Movement
- Flex your elbows to raise the bar in an arc toward your shoulders.
- Keep your upper arms pressed against your torso during the exercise.

### Downward Movement
- Allow your elbows to extend to the initial position.
- Lower the bar in an arc until your elbows are fully extended.

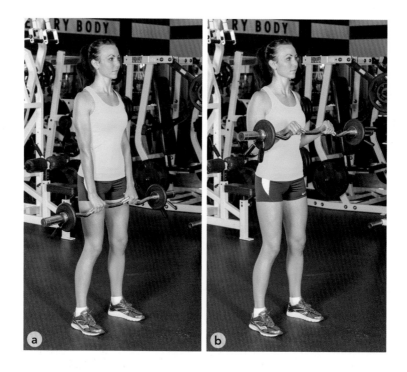

# LOW-PULLEY CURL*

**EXERCISE TYPE:** machine (pulley)

**MAJOR MUSCLE TRAINED:** biceps brachii

## Initial Position

- Stand in front (or sit in the attached seat) of a low-pulley station.
- Grasp the bar using a closed, supinated grip shoulder-width apart.
- Slightly flex your knees and position the bar in front of your thighs with your elbows fully extended.

## Upward Movement

- Flex your elbows to raise the bar in an arc toward your shoulders.
- Keep your upper arms pressed against your torso during the exercise.

## Downward Movement

- Allow your elbows to extend to the initial position.
- Lower the bar in an arc until your elbows are fully extended.

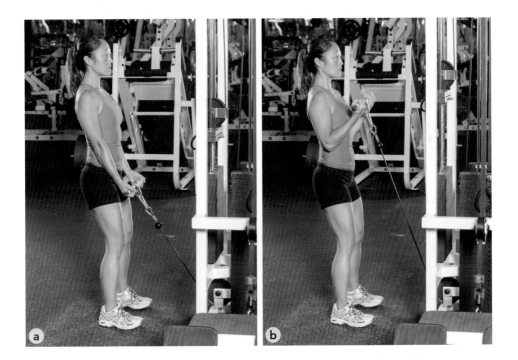

## PREACHER CURL*

**EXERCISE TYPE:** machine (cam)

**MAJOR MUSCLE TRAINED:** biceps brachii

### Initial Position

- Sit in the machine, press your chest against the pad, and place your feet flat on the floor.
- Grasp the handles using a closed, supinated grip with your elbows fully extended.
- Move your upper arms on the arm pad to be parallel with each other with your elbows lined up with the axis of the machine.

### Upward Movement

- Flex your elbows to raise the handles in an arc toward your shoulders.
- Keep your chest and upper arms pressed against the pads.

### Downward Movement

- Allow your elbows to extend to the initial position.
- Lower the handles in an arc until your elbows are fully extended.

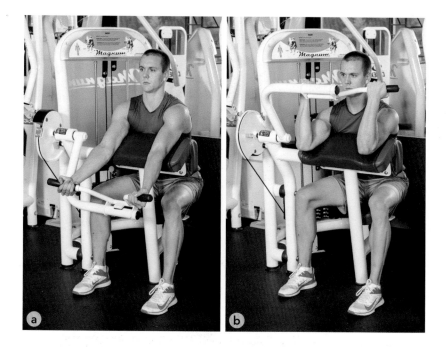

## BICEPS CURL (DB)

**EXERCISE TYPE:** alternative

**MAJOR MUSCLE TRAINED:** biceps brachii

### Initial Position
- Grasp two dumbbells using a closed, neutral grip.
- Stand with your knees slightly flexed and the dumbbells positioned at the sides of your thighs with your elbows fully extended.

### Upward Movement
- Flex your right elbow to raise the dumbbell upward in an arc, turning the palm up as the dumbbell moves closer to your right shoulder.
- Keep the upper part of your right arm pressed against your torso.
- Keep your left arm stationary at your side.

### Downward Movement
- Allow your right elbow to extend to the initial position.
- Lower the dumbbell in an arc until your right elbow is fully extended.
- Repeat the exercise with your left arm and continue by alternating arms.

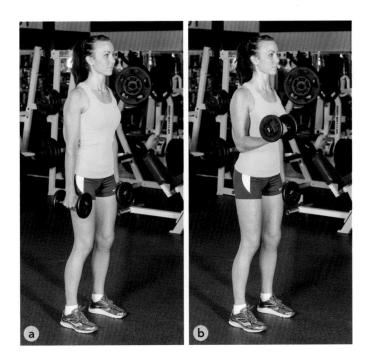

## BICEPS CURL (RB)

**EXERCISE TYPE:** alternative

**MAJOR MUSCLE TRAINED:** biceps brachii

### Initial Position

- Grasp the handles of the band with a closed, supinated grip.
- Stand on top of the middle of the band with your feet shoulder-width apart.
- Move your arms and handles to the outside of your thighs with your palms facing forward with your elbows fully extended.

### Upward Movement

- Flex your elbows to raise the handles in an arc toward your shoulders.
- Keep your body erect with your knees slightly flexed and feet flat on the floor.

### Downward Movement

- Allow your elbows to extend to move the handles down to the initial position.
- Lower the handles in an arc until your elbows are fully extended.
- Keep your body erect with your knees slightly flexed and feet flat on the floor.

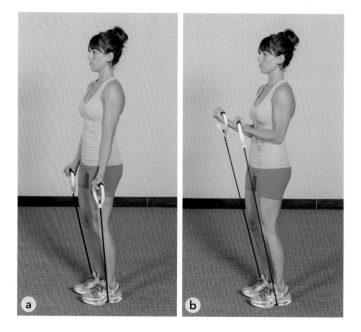

# HAMMER CURL (DB)

**EXERCISE TYPE: alternative**

**MAJOR MUSCLE TRAINED: biceps brachii**

### Initial Position
- Grasp two dumbbells using a closed, neutral grip.
- Stand with your knees slightly flexed and the dumbbells positioned at the sides of your thighs with your elbows fully extended.

### Upward Movement
- Flex your right elbow to raise the dumbbell upward in an arc, keeping the dumbbell in a neutral position during the exercise.
- Keep the upper part of your right arm pressed against your torso.
- Keep your left arm stationary at your side.

### Downward Movement
- Allow your right elbow to extend to the initial position.
- Lower the dumbbell in an arc until your right elbow is fully extended.
- Repeat the exercise with your left arm and continue by alternating arms.

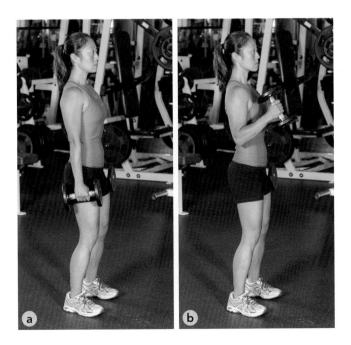

# BACK OF ARMS (TRICEPS)

## LYING TRICEPS EXTENSION*

**EXERCISE TYPE:** barbell

**MAJOR MUSCLE TRAINED:** triceps brachii

✋ **IMPORTANT:** A spotter is recommended!

### Initial Position

- Lie faceup on a bench with your head, back, and buttocks in contact with the bench and your feet flat on the floor.
- Take the bar from the spotter with a closed, pronated grip about shoulder-width (or slightly narrower) apart.
- Hold the bar over your chest with your elbows extended.

### Downward Movement

- Allow your elbows to flex to lower the bar in an arc to almost touch the top of your head (depending on the length of your arms).
- Keep your upper arms parallel to each other; do not let your elbows flare out as you lower the bar.
- Keep your head, back, and buttocks in contact with the bench and your feet flat on the floor.

### Upward Movement

- Extend your elbows to move the bar in an arc to the initial position.
- Keep your upper arms parallel to each other and perpendicular to the floor.
- Keep your head, back, and buttocks in contact with the bench and your feet flat on the floor.
- When you complete the set, allow the spotter to take the bar from your hands.

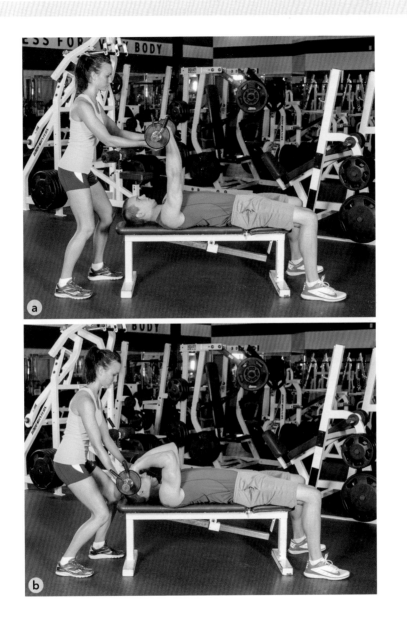

## SEATED OVERHEAD TRICEPS EXTENSION

**EXERCISE TYPE:** barbell

**MAJOR MUSCLE TRAINED:** triceps brachii

**IMPORTANT:** A spotter is recommended!

### Initial Position

- Grasp the bar with a closed, pronated grip about shoulder-width (or slightly narrower) apart.
- Sit erect on a shoulder press bench with your head, upper back, and hips pressed against the pads. If one is not available, you can straddle a flat bench, but be sure to sit in an erect position with your feet flat on the floor.
- Move the bar to position it over your head with your palms facing forward.

### Downward Movement

- Allow your elbows to flex to lower the bar down in an arc behind your head.
- Keep your upper arms parallel to each other; do not let your elbows flare out as you lower the bar.
- Maintain your erect torso position with your feet flat on the floor.

### Upward Movement

- Extend your elbows to move the bar in an arc to the initial position.
- Keep your upper arms parallel to each other and perpendicular to the floor.
- Maintain your erect torso position; do not lean back or lift off the bench as you extend your elbows.
- When you complete the set, allow the spotter to take the bar from your hands.

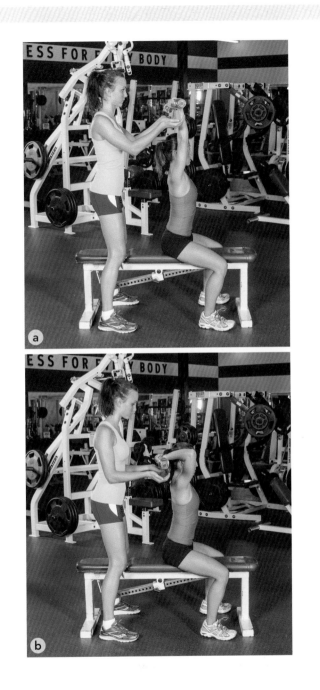

**EXERCISE TYPE:** machine (cam)

**MAJOR MUSCLE TRAINED:** triceps brachii

### Initial Position

- Sit in the machine, press your back against the pad, and place your feet flat on the floor.
- If there is a seat belt, secure it across your upper thighs.
- Grasp the handles using a closed, neutral grip with your elbows flexed and your arms near the sides of your torso.

### Downward Movement

- Push the handles down until your elbows are fully extended.
- Keep your back and upper arms pressed against the pads.

### Upward Movement

- Allow your elbows to flex to the initial position.

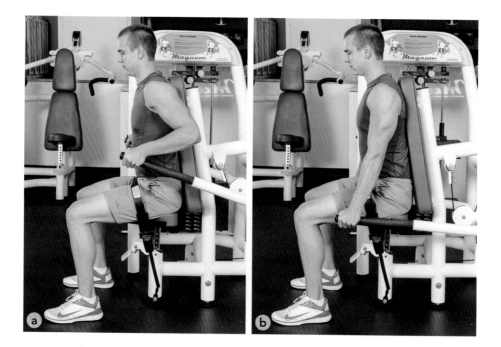

# ONE-ARM TRICEPS EXTENSION (RB)

**EXERCISE TYPE:** alternative

**MAJOR MUSCLE TRAINED:** triceps brachii

### Initial Position
- Grasp the handles of the band with a closed, pronated grip.
- Sit erect on the floor with your legs out in front of you with your knees flexed to position your feet flat on the floor.
- Position your body and the band so that you are sitting on top of the middle of the band.
- Flex your elbows to move your arms and handles behind your head and upper back with your palms facing forward.

### Upward Movement
- Extend your right elbow until your hand is over your head.
- Do not let your wrist flex, and keep your upper arm next to your head.
- Keep the left arm stationary as the right elbow extends.

### Downward Movement
- Allow your right elbow to flex to move the handle down to the initial position.
- Repeat the exercise with your left arm and continue by alternating arms.

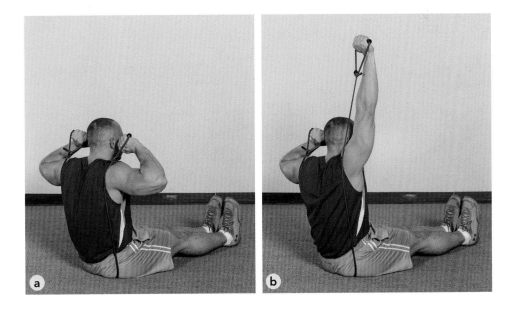

## TRICEPS PUSHDOWN*

**EXERCISE TYPE: machine (pulley)**

**MAJOR MUSCLE TRAINED: triceps brachii**

### Initial Position

- Face the machine and stand next to the hanging bar.
- Grasp the bar with a closed, pronated grip slightly narrower than shoulder width.
- Place your feet shoulder-width apart with your knees slightly flexed.
- Pull the bar down and place your upper arms against the sides of your torso with your forearms slightly above parallel with the floor.
- Stand erect with the cable in front of your nose.

### Downward Movement

- Push the bar down until your elbows are fully extended.
- Keep the rest of your body stationary with your upper arms next to your torso.

### Upward Movement

- Allow your elbows to flex to the initial position.
- Keep your upper arms next to your torso.
- When you complete the set, raise your arms up to set the weight back down to its resting position.

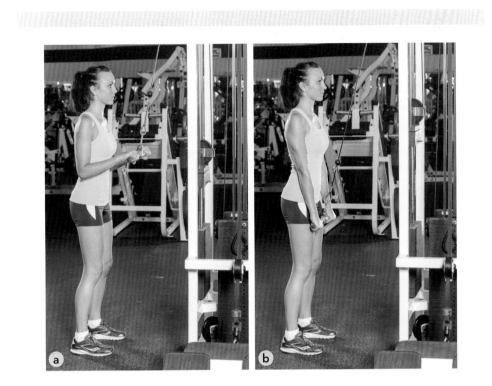

103

## TRICEPS KICKBACK (DB)

**EXERCISE TYPE: alternative**

**MAJOR MUSCLE TRAINED: triceps brachii**

### Initial Position

- Set one dumbbell on the floor on the right side of the bench.
- Stand on the right side of a flat bench and kneel on the bench with your left leg.
- Flex forward and position your left hand on the bench in front of your left knee so that your left arm and left thigh are approximately parallel to each other.
- Slightly flex your right knee and hold this position during the exercise.
- Reach down and pick up a dumbbell with your right hand using a closed, neutral grip.
- Lift the dumbbell up and flex your right elbow 90 degrees to position the upper part of your right arm next to your torso with the dumbbell hanging straight down from your elbow.

### Upward Movement

- Extend your right elbow until your arm is straight and parallel to the floor.
- Keep the upper part of your right arm against your torso as you extend your elbow.
- Keep your right wrist straight.
- Keep the rest of your body stationary.

### Downward Movement

- Allow your right elbow to flex to lower the dumbbell to the initial position.
- Keep the rest of your body stationary.
- When you complete the set, set the dumbbell on the floor and then stand on the left side of the bench. Repeat the movement with your left arm.

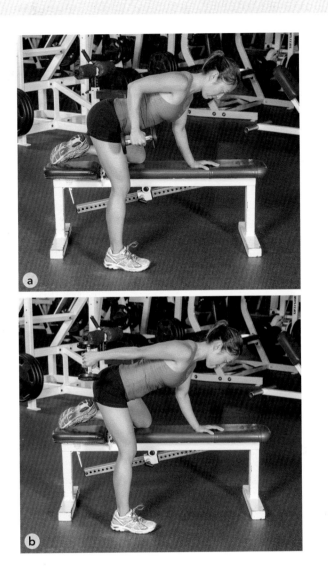

# THIGH

## LUNGE

**EXERCISE TYPE: barbell**

**MAJOR MUSCLES TRAINED: gluteus maximus, hamstrings, quadriceps**

✋ **IMPORTANT:** A spotter is recommended!

### Initial Position

- If the bar is in a rack, step under the middle of the bar and position your feet parallel to each other directly under the bar. Grasp the bar with a closed, pronated grip slightly wider than shoulder width. Dip under the bar and position your body so that you can place the bar evenly on your upper back at the base of your neck and across the back of your shoulders.
- If you have to lift the bar off the floor, follow the guidelines for the power clean exercise first, then the guidelines for the standing press exercise to move the bar over your head. Then, instead of lowering the bar down to the front of your shoulders, lower it to be positioned on your upper back at the base of your neck and across your shoulders.
- Once the bar is in position, move your shoulders back and your chest out so your back is flat and your torso is erect.
- Position your feet approximately shoulder-width apart with your toes pointed straight ahead.
- If the bar began in a rack, extend your hips and knees to lift the bar off the racks, take two steps backward, and then reposition your feet approximately shoulder-width apart. See photo a.

### Forward Movement

- Take one exaggerated step directly ahead with your left foot.
- Keep your right leg and foot in the initial position but allow your right knee to flex as you step forward.
- Place your left foot squarely on the floor with your toes pointing straight ahead or slightly inward. See photo b.
- When both feet are in firm contact with the floor (your whole left foot and the ball of your right foot), flex your left knee to lower your right knee toward the floor.
- Allow your left hip and knee to flex as you lunge forward and down.
- Continue lunging until your right knee is close to the floor but not touching it.

- Be sure that your left knee does not flex past the toes of your left foot.
- Do not lean forward as you lunge; if you hold your shoulders back and keep your chest out, you can more easily maintain the correct torso position. See photo c.

**Backward Movement**
- Push off the floor by extending your left hip and knee. Your right hip and knee will extend also.
- Continue to move backward (do not stutter step) to the initial position. See photo a.
- Keep your torso erect and the bar firmly on your shoulders.
- For your next repetition, step forward with your right leg.
- Alternate legs with each repetition.

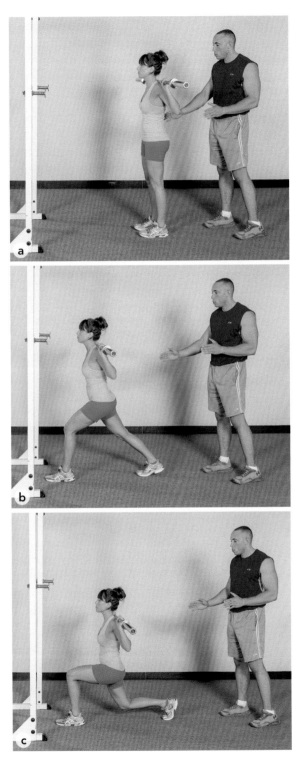

## SQUAT

**EXERCISE TYPE: barbell**

**MAJOR MUSCLES TRAINED: gluteus maximus, hamstrings, quadriceps**

✋ **IMPORTANT:** At least one spotter is recommended!

### Initial Position

- Step under the middle of the bar and position your feet parallel to each other directly under the bar. Grasp the bar with a closed, pronated grip slightly wider than shoulder width. Dip under the bar and position your body so that you can place the bar evenly on your upper back at the base of your neck and across the back of your shoulders.
- Move your shoulders back and your chest out so your back is flat and your torso is erect.
- Position your feet approximately shoulder-width apart with your toes pointed straight ahead. See photo *a*.
- Extend your hips and knees to lift the bar off the racks, stand erect, take a half of a step backward, and then reposition your feet approximately shoulder-width apart with your toes pointed slightly outward rather than straight ahead. See photo *b*.

### Downward Movement

- Allow your hips and knees to flex at the same rate to keep the near-erect flat-back torso position.
- Do not lean forward as you squat down; if you hold your shoulders back and keep your chest out, you can more easily keep the correct torso position.
- Keep your heels in full contact with the floor and your knees aligned over your feet.
- Continue the downward movement until your thighs are approximately parallel to the floor (but if your heels lift off the floor or you begin to lean forward, you squatted down too far; perform your remaining repetitions with a shallower squat). See photo *c*.

### Upward Movement

- Extend your hips and knees at the same rate to stand back up to the initial position. See photo *b*.
- Keep your back flat, heels on the floor, and knees aligned over your feet.

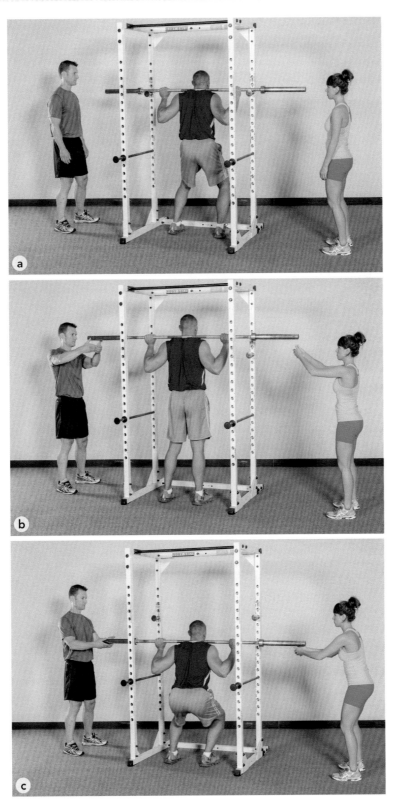

**EXERCISE TYPE: machine**

**MAJOR MUSCLES TRAINED: gluteus maximus, hamstrings, quadriceps**

### Initial Position

- Sit in the machine with your head, back, and buttocks in contact with the pads.
- Position your feet hip-width apart and in the middle of the foot platform.
- Position your legs parallel to each other.
- Grasp the handles or the side of the seat.
- Slightly extend your hips and knees to lift the foot platform so that you can move the support bar out of the way.
- Regrasp the handles or the side of the seat and fully extend your hips and knees.

### Downward Movement

- Allow your hips and knees to flex at the same rate to keep your back and buttocks in contact with the pads.
- Keep your heels in full contact with the foot platform and your knees aligned with your feet.
- Continue the downward movement until your thighs are parallel to the foot platform. (But if your heels lift off the platform or your hips or buttocks lose contact with the seat, you allowed the platform to go down too low; perform your remaining repetitions within a smaller range of motion.)

### Upward Movement

- Extend your hips and knees at the same rate to push the foot platform back up to the initial position.
- Keep your heels in full contact with the foot platform and your knees aligned with your feet.
- When you complete the set, move the support bar back into place and step out of the machine.

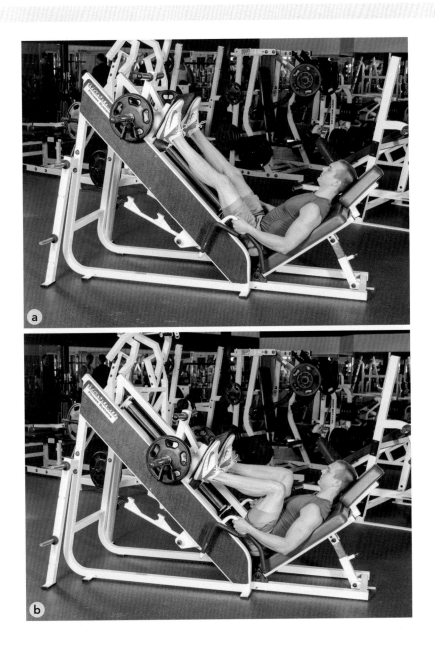

## LEG PRESS*

**EXERCISE TYPE: machine**

**MAJOR MUSCLES TRAINED: gluteus maximus, hamstrings, quadriceps**

### Initial Position

- Lie or sit in the machine with your back and buttocks in contact with the pads.
- Position your feet hip-width apart and in the middle of the foot platform. If possible, change the seat position or the foot platform so that your thighs are parallel to the foot platform in the initial position.
- Position your legs parallel to each other.
- Grasp the handles or the sides of the seat.

### Forward Movement

- Extend your hips and knees to push the foot pedals away from you. (Some machines may have a fixed foot platform with a seat that moves you backward.)
- Keep your heels in full contact with the foot pedals, your knees aligned with your feet, and your back and buttocks in contact with the pads.
- Continue to push the foot platform forward until your knees are fully extended.

### Backward Movement

- Allow your hips and knees to flex to return the foot pedals to the initial position.
- Keep your back and buttocks in contact with the pads.

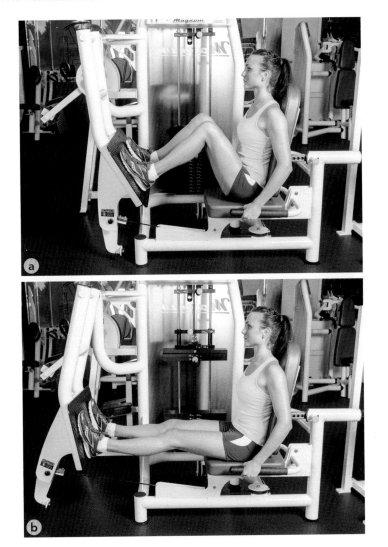

113

## FRONT SQUAT (KB)

**EXERCISE TYPE:** alternative

**MAJOR MUSCLES TRAINED:** gluteus maximus, hamstrings, quadriceps

### Initial Position

- Stand erect and hold a kettlebell at the front of your shoulders (either one in each hand or one held with both hands); if you keep your elbows up, you can more easily hold the kettlebell next to your shoulders.
- Move your shoulders back and your chest out so your back is flat and your torso is erect.
- Position your feet approximately shoulder-width apart with your toes pointed slightly outward.

### Downward Movement

- Allow your hips and knees to flex at the same rate to keep your torso erect and back flat.
- Do not lean forward as you squat down; keep your shoulders back and your chest out with the kettlebell in the same position at the front of your shoulders.
- Keep your heels in full contact with the floor and your knees aligned over your feet.
- Continue the downward movement until your thighs are parallel to the floor. (But if your heels lift off the floor or you begin to lean forward, you squatted down too far; perform your remaining repetitions with a shallower squat.)

### Upward Movement

- Extend your hips and knees at the same rate to stand back up to the initial position.
- Keep your back flat, heels on the floor, and knees aligned over your feet.

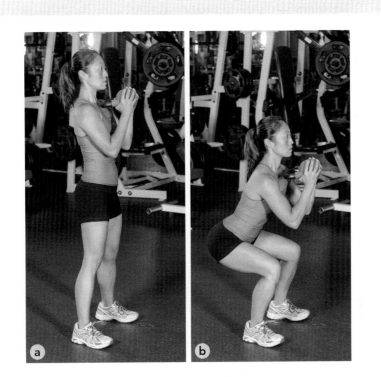

## LUNGE (DB)*

**EXERCISE TYPE:** alternative

**MAJOR MUSCLES TRAINED: gluteus maximus, hamstrings, quadriceps**

### Initial Position

- Grasp two dumbbells using a closed, neutral grip.
- Stand erect with the dumbbells positioned at the sides of your thighs and your elbows extended.
- Move your shoulders back and your chest out so your back is flat and your torso is erect.
- Position your feet approximately shoulder-width apart with your toes pointed straight ahead.

### Forward Movement

- Take one exaggerated step directly ahead with your left foot.
- Keep your right leg and foot in the initial position but allow your right knee to flex as you step forward.
- Place the left foot squarely on the floor with your toes pointing straight ahead or slightly inward.
- When both feet are in firm contact with the floor (your whole left foot and the ball of your right foot), flex your left knee to lower your right knee toward the floor.
- Allow your left hip and knee to flex as you lunge forward and down.
- Continue lunging until your right knee is close to the floor but not touching it.
- Be sure that your left knee does not flex past the toes of your left foot.
- Do not lean forward as you lunge.
- Keep both arms and dumbbells hanging straight down at your sides during the exercise; be careful not to hit your thighs with the dumbbells.

### Backward Movement

- Push off the floor by extending your left hip and knee. Your right hip and knee will extend also.
- Continue to move backward (do not stutter step) to the initial position.
- Keep your torso erect.
- Do not let the dumbbells swing backward as you perform the exercise.
- For your next repetition, step forward with your right leg.
- Alternate legs with each repetition.

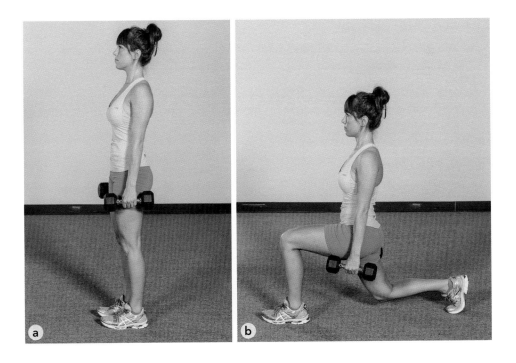

**EXERCISE TYPE:** alternative

**MAJOR MUSCLES TRAINED:** gluteus maximus, hamstrings, quadriceps

### Initial Position

- Grasp two dumbbells using a closed, neutral grip.
- Stand erect with the dumbbells positioned at the sides of your thighs and your elbows extended.
- Move your shoulders back and your chest out so your back is flat and your torso is erect.
- Position your feet approximately shoulder-width apart with your toes pointed slightly outward.

### Downward Movement

- Allow your hips and knees to flex at the same rate to keep the near-erect flat-back torso position.
- Do not lean forward as you squat down.
- Keep your heels in full contact with the floor and your knees aligned over your feet.
- Keep both arms and dumbbells hanging straight down at your sides during the exercise.
- Continue the downward movement until your thighs are approximately parallel to the floor. (But if your heels lift off the floor or you begin to lean forward, you squatted down too far; perform your remaining repetitions with a shallower squat.)

### Upward Movement

- Extend your hips and knees at the same rate to stand back up to the initial position.
- Keep your back flat, heels on the floor, and knees aligned over your feet.

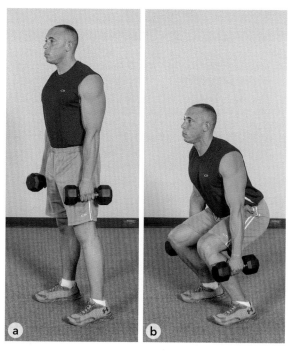

## SQUAT (RB)

**EXERCISE TYPE:** alternative

**MAJOR MUSCLES TRAINED:** gluteus maximus, hamstrings, quadriceps

### Initial Position

- Grasp the handles of the band with a closed, pronated grip.
- Stand on top of the middle of the band with your feet shoulder- or hip-width apart.
- Squat down so that your thighs are not lower than parallel to the floor.
- Gather the extra slack of the resistance band between your feet so the band is taut.
- Move your shoulders back and your chest out so your back is flat, not rounded.
- Move your arms to position the handles to the outside of your shoulders with your palms facing upward.

### Upward Movement

- Extend your hips and knees at the same rate until you are fully standing.
- Keep your heels in full contact with the floor and your knees aligned over your feet.

### Downward Movement

- Allow your hips and knees to flex at the same rate to the initial position.
- Keep your heels in full contact with the floor and your knees aligned over your feet.

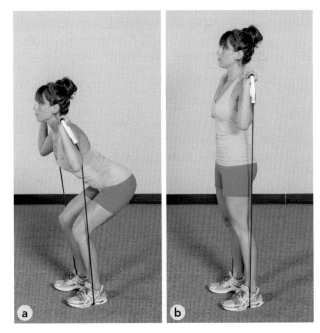

## STEP-UP (DB)

**EXERCISE TYPE:** alternative

**MAJOR MUSCLES TRAINED:** gluteus maximus, hamstrings, quadriceps

### Initial Position

*Note:* The box should be 12 to 18 inches (30-46 cm) high, or high enough to create a 90-degree angle at your knee when your foot is on the box.

- Grasp two dumbbells using a closed, neutral grip.
- Walk toward the box and stand in a position near the box that is as far away from the box as the box is tall.
- Stand erect with the dumbbells positioned at the sides of your thighs and your elbows extended.
- Move your shoulders back and your chest out so your back is flat and your torso is erect.
- Position your feet approximately shoulder-width apart with your toes pointed straight ahead.

### Upward Movement

- Step up with your left foot and place your entire foot on the top of the box. See photo *a*.
- Keep your right foot in the initial position, but shift your body weight to your left leg.
- Forcefully extend your left hip and knee to move your body to a standing position on top of the box. See photo *b*.
- Do not push off or hop up with your right leg or foot.
- Keep both arms and dumbbells hanging straight down at your sides during the exercise; be careful not to hit your thighs with the dumbbells.
- At the highest position, stand erect and pause before beginning the downward movement. See photo *c*.

### Downward Movement

- Shift your body weight to your left leg.
- Step off the box with your right leg. See photo *b*.
- Keep your torso erect; do not lean forward.
- Place your right foot on the floor 12 to 18 inches (30-46 cm) away from the box. See photo *a*.
- When your right foot is in full contact with the floor, shift your body weight to your right leg.

- Step off the box with your left foot.
- Bring your left foot to a position next to your right foot.
- Do not let the dumbbells swing backward as you step down.
- Stand erect and pause in the initial position before beginning the next repetition.
- For your next repetition, step up with your right foot.
- Alternate legs with each repetition.

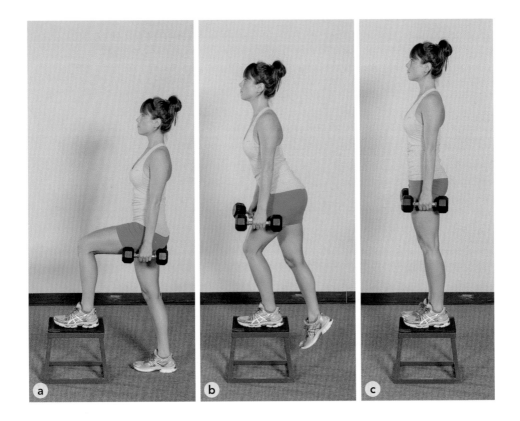

## LEG (KNEE) CURL

**EXERCISE TYPE:** machine

**MAJOR MUSCLES TRAINED:** hamstrings

### Initial Position

- Move the thigh pad to its highest position.
- Sit in the machine with your back and thighs positioned in the seat so that your knees are aligned with the axis of the machine.
- Position your heels on top of the ankle pad with the lower part of your calf or back of your heels pressing against the pad.
- Adjust the thigh pad so it is firmly pressed against your thighs just above the knees.
- Be sure that your thighs, lower legs, and feet are parallel to each other.
- Grasp the handles or the sides of the torso pad.

### Upward Movement

- Flex your knees until the ankle pad nearly touches the base of the machine.
- Keep your thighs, lower legs, and feet parallel to each other.
- Keep the rest of your body stationary.

### Downward Movement

- Allow your knees to extend to the initial position.
- Keep your thighs, lower legs, and feet parallel to each other.
- Keep the rest of your body stationary.

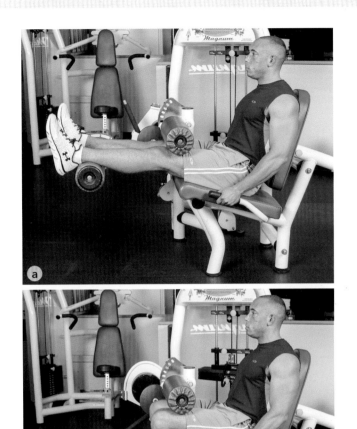

# LEG CURL (HEEL PULL) (SB)

**EXERCISE TYPE:** alternative

**MAJOR MUSCLES TRAINED:** hamstrings

### Initial Position
- Lie faceup on the floor with your body straight, hips lifted off the floor, and lower calves and back of heels on the top of a stability ball.
- Move your arms out from your torso with your palms facing the floor.

### Backward Movement
- Keeping your upper body in the same position, flex your knees to move your heels toward your buttocks to roll the stability ball backward (toward you).
- Continue flexing your knees until they are at a 90-degree angle and the soles of your feet are nearly flat near the top of the stability ball.
- Keep your knees, hips, and torso in a straight line.

### Forward Movement
- Extend your knees to roll the ball forward to the initial position.
- Keep your hips lifted throughout the exercise.

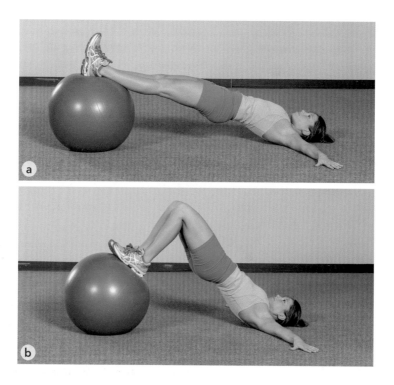

## LEG (KNEE) EXTENSION

**EXERCISE TYPE: machine**

**MAJOR MUSCLES TRAINED: quadriceps**

### Initial Position
- Sit in the machine with your back and thighs positioned in the seat so that your knees are aligned with the axis of the machine.
- Position your feet under the ankle pad with the insteps of your feet pressing against the pad.
- Be sure that your thighs, lower legs, and feet are parallel to each other.
- Grasp the handles or the sides of the seat.

### Upward Movement
- Extend your knees until they are straight.
- Keep your thighs, lower legs, and feet parallel to each other.
- Keep the rest of your body stationary.

### Downward Movement
- Allow your knees to flex to the initial position.
- Keep your thighs, lower legs, and feet parallel to each other.
- Keep the rest of your body stationary.

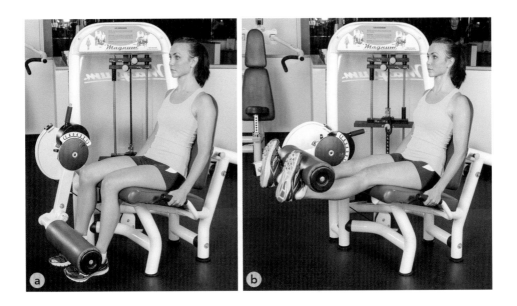

## WALL SQUAT (SB)

**EXERCISE TYPE: alternative**

**MAJOR MUSCLES TRAINED: quadriceps**

### Initial Position

- Position a stability ball between an empty wall and your lower back.
- Lean back to put pressure on the stability ball and shuffle your feet to position them 12 to 18 inches (30-46 cm) in front of you and wider than shoulder-width apart.
- Move your shoulders back and your chest out so your back is flat and your torso is erect.
- Cross your arms in front of your chest.

### Downward Movement

- While leaning back to keep pressure on the stability ball, allow your hips and knees to flex at the same rate to roll the ball down the wall.
- Keep your shoulders back and your chest out with your heels in full contact with the floor and your knees aligned over your feet.
- Continue the downward movement until your thighs are parallel to the floor.

### Upward Movement

- Extend your hips and knees at the same rate to stand back up to the initial position.
- Keep pressure on the stability ball to roll the ball up the wall.
- Keep your back flat, heels on the floor, and knees aligned over your feet.

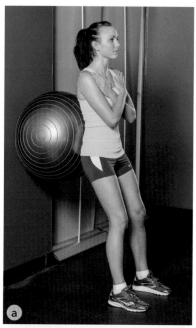

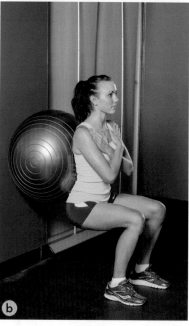

## SEATED HEEL RAISE

**EXERCISE TYPE:** machine

**MAJOR MUSCLES TRAINED: soleus, gastrocnemius**

### Initial Position

- Sit in the machine and place your knees and thighs under the pads.
- Position the balls of your feet on the closest edge of the step with your feet parallel to each other.
- Point your toes slightly to lift the thigh pads so that you can move the support bar out of the way.
- Allow your heels to drop down lower than the step until you feel a stretch.

### Upward Movement

- Point your toes to lift your heels up.
- Do not pull on the handles or lean your torso backward.

### Downward Movement

- Allow your heels to drop back down to the initial position.
- When you complete the set, move the support bar back into place.

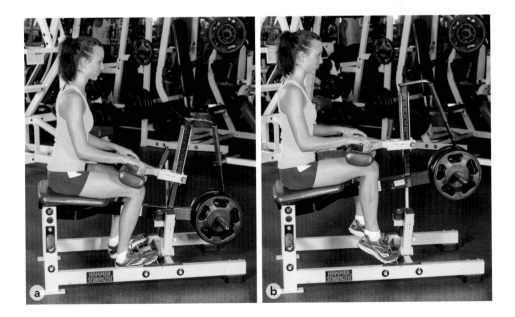

**EXERCISE TYPE: machine**

**MAJOR MUSCLES TRAINED: soleus, gastrocnemius**

### Initial Position

- Face the machine and place the balls of your feet on the closest edge of the step with your feet parallel to each other.
- Dip your body under the shoulder pads and stand up with your body fully erect.
- Allow your heels to drop down lower than the step until you feel a stretch.
- Do not allow your knees to be locked out.

### Upward Movement

- Point your toes to lift your heels up.
- Keep your body erect and do not look down or lean forward or backward.

### Downward Movement

- Allow your heels to drop back down to the initial position.
- Keep your body fully erect and do not bounce up from the lowest position to begin the upward movement.

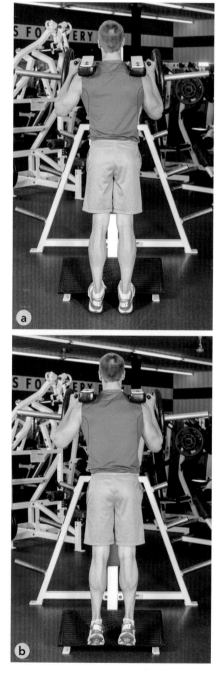

## ONE-LEG STANDING HEEL RAISE (DB)

**EXERCISE TYPE:** alternative

**MAJOR MUSCLES TRAINED:** soleus, gastrocnemius

### Initial Position

- Grasp a dumbbell with your left hand and allow it to hang at your side.
- Place the ball of your left foot on the closest edge of a step, platform, or board with your right foot hooked around the back of your left leg.
- With your right hand, hold on to a railing or wall edge for balance.
- Allow your left heel to drop down lower than the step, platform, or board until you feel a stretch.
- Do not allow your left knee to be locked out.

### Upward Movement

- Point the toes of your left foot to lift your left heel up.
- Keep your body erect and do not look down or lean forward or backward.

### Downward Movement

- Allow your left heel to drop back down to the initial position.
- Keep your body erect and do not bounce up from the lowest position to begin the upward movement.
- When you complete the set, grasp the dumbbell with your right hand and repeat the movement with your right foot.

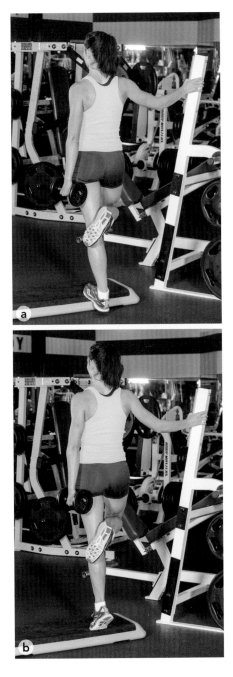

129

## POWER CLEAN

**EXERCISE TYPE:** barbell

**MAJOR MUSCLES TRAINED:** gluteus maximus, hamstrings, quadriceps, soleus, gastrocnemius, deltoids, trapezius

### Initial Position

- Stand with your feet hip-width apart with your toes pointed slightly outward.
- Squat down with your hips lower than your shoulders and grasp the bar with a closed, pronated grip about shoulder-width apart, outside your knees, with your elbows fully extended.
- Place your feet flat on the floor and position the bar over the balls of your feet.
- Position your back so that it is flat and tilt your head slightly backward. See photo a.

### Upward Movement: First Pull

- Rapidly extend your hips and knees at the same rate to keep the near-erect flat-back position and the bar close to your shins.
- Keep your heels in full contact with the floor and your knees aligned over your feet.
- Keep your elbows fully extended and your shoulders over or slightly ahead of the bar. See photo b.

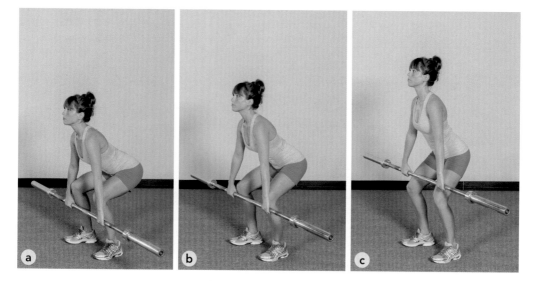

### Upward Movement: Scoop (Transition)

- As the bar rises just above your knees, move your hips forward and quickly flex your knees to move them under the bar.
- Keep the near-erect torso and flat-back position with your elbows still fully extended. See photo c.

### Upward Movement: Second Pull

- Immediately after your knees move under the bar, rapidly jump up by extending your hips and knees and pointing your feet.
- Keep the bar near your body and maintain the near-erect torso and flat-back position with your elbows still extended.
- After you fully extend your hips, knees, and ankles, rapidly shrug your shoulders with your elbows still extended. See photo d.
- After you fully shrug your shoulders, flex your elbows to continue moving the bar upward.

### Upward Movement: Catch

- After the bar reaches its maximum height, rotate your arms around and then under the bar and, at the same time, flex your hips and knees into a quarter-squat position.
- Catch the bar at the front of your shoulders. Be sure that your torso is in a flat-back position when you catch the bar. See photo e.
- After you catch the bar, stand up by extending your hips and knees. See photo f.

### Downward Movement

- Reverse your arm and leg movements to allow the bar to move back down first to your thighs and then to the initial position on the floor.

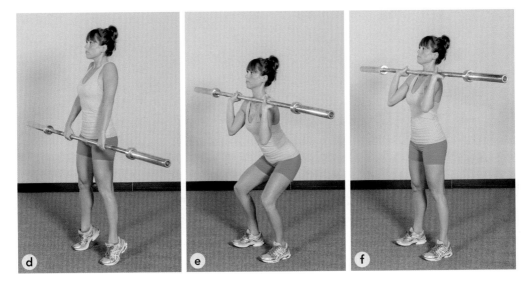

**EXERCISE TYPE:** barbell

**MAJOR MUSCLES TRAINED:** gluteus maximus, hamstrings, quadriceps, soleus, gastrocnemius, deltoids, trapezius

### Initial Position

- Stand with your feet hip-width apart with your toes pointed slightly outward.
- Squat down with your hips lower than your shoulders and grasp the bar with a closed, pronated grip about shoulder-width apart, outside your knees, with your elbows fully extended.
- Place your feet flat on the floor and position the bar over the balls of your feet.
- Position your back so that it is flat and tilt your head slightly backward.
- Follow all of the guidelines for upward movement of the power clean exercise to lift the bar off the floor to your shoulders. See photo a.

### Upward Movement: Dip

- Flex your hips and knees at a slow to moderate speed to move the bar in a straight path downward. Do not dip more than approximately 8 inches (20 cm).
- Keep your torso erect and head in neutral position. See photo b.

### Upward Movement: Drive

- Immediately after reaching the lowest position of the dip, rapidly reverse the movement by fully extending your knees and hips to jump straight up.

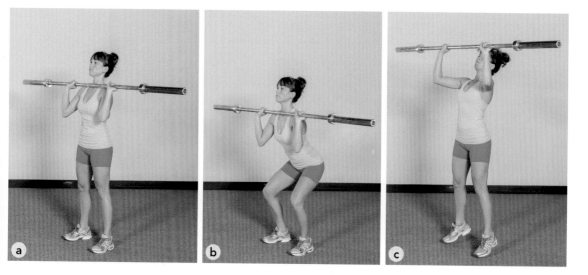

- Tip your head back slightly to allow the bar to pass by your chin; as it does, start pushing the bar up with your arms. See photo c.
- Keep your torso erect so the bar is pushed directly over your head, not forward or backward.

### Upward Movement: Catch
- When the bar is directly overhead, catch it with your elbows fully extended.
- At the same time, slightly flex your knees and hips to absorb the bar's weight.
- Keep your torso erect and eyes focused forward. After the bar is balanced overhead, stand up to a fully erect position by extending your hips and knees. See photo d.

### Downward Movement
- Allow the bar to lower to your shoulders.
- Slightly flex your knees and hips to absorb the weight.
- Keep your torso erect and eyes focused forward. See photo e.
- Continue the dip, drive, and downward movements until the set is complete; do not set the bar back down on the floor between repetitions.
- When you complete the set, pause and lower the bar to your thighs. Keep the bar close to your chest and abdomen as it lowers.
- From your thighs, allow the bar to lower past your knees and to the floor using a squatting movement.

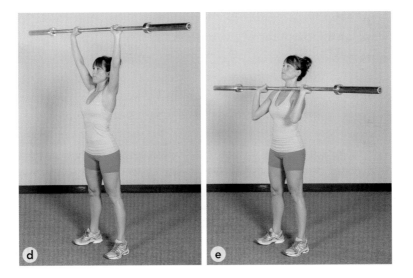

## SWING (KB)

**EXERCISE TYPE: alternative**

**MAJOR MUSCLES TRAINED: gluteus maximus, hamstrings, quadriceps**

### Initial Position

- Straddle a kettlebell with your feet moderately wider than shoulder-width apart with your toes pointed slightly outward.
- Squat down with your torso erect and grasp a kettlebell with both hands side by side using a closed, pronated grip.
- Stand up with the kettlebell and allow it to hang between your legs with your elbows fully extended.
- Move with your shoulders back and your chest out so your torso is erect. See photo a.

### Forward and Upward Movement

- To cause the kettlebell to start moving, squat down and use a small effort of your arms to move the kettlebell back between your legs. (For the rest of the exercise, your arms do not play an active role to move the kettlebell.)
- At the bottom of the swing, your forearms (with your elbows fully extended) are pressed against your inner thighs, and the kettlebell can be seen behind your calves. See photo b.
- To cause the kettlebell to move forward and up, simultaneously squat up and thrust your hips forward.
- Keep your shoulders back and your chest out.
- Guide the kettlebell up with your elbows still fully extended until the kettlebell reaches approximately shoulder or face height. See photo c.

### Backward and Downward Movement

- After the kettlebell reaches its highest position, allow it to lower under control down to its lowest position with your arms extended.
- As the kettlebell lowers to the bottom of its swing, squat down slightly with your hips and shoulders back, chest out, and forearms pressed against your inner thighs. See photo b.
- When you complete the set, allow the kettlebell to swing forward, but do not extend your hips and knees to continue the swing.
- After a few repetitions when the swing has stopped, place the kettlebell on the floor between your feet.

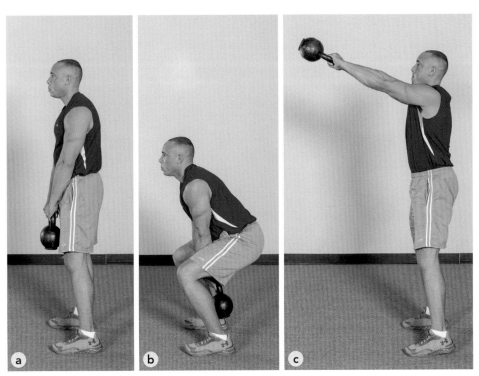

# Part II

# Training by the Color Zones

Up to this point, you have learned about the contributions and outcomes of a weight training program, common gear and equipment, your current training status and desired goal, and the steps involved in setting up your program. What is missing? Yes, the actual program you will follow!

This section is organized into six color-coded workout zones, one per chapter. Each of the 75 workout charts is placed in a zone according to its level of difficulty. Green Zone workouts are the easiest and take the shortest time to complete, followed by the Blue, Purple, Yellow, and Orange Zone workouts; Red Zone workouts are the most difficult and take the most time to complete. In each of the zones, you will have an opportunity to select workouts that improve muscle toning, body shaping, or muscular strength.

## Understanding the Workout Zones

Each workout table in chapters 7 to 12 provides the following information:

- The training goal, color zone, and workout number.
- The total time it will take to complete the workout, including the warm-up and cool-down periods.
- The number of weeks and the number of days per week that you will complete the workout. For example, you should perform the Green Zone muscle toning workout 1 for two weeks at a rate of two nonconsecutive training sessions per week.
- A description of the weight training session in detail, including the muscle group trained by each exercise, the recommended number of repetitions and sets for each exercise, and three columns of exercises (each is a different type). As explained in chapter 4, you will choose one exercise (not all three) for each of the seven major muscle groups: chest, back, shoulders, front of upper arm (biceps), back of upper arm

(triceps), thighs, and core. Higher-intensity workouts include more exercises that train these muscles. If you have never performed a certain exercise or if you are unsure about the correct technique for an exercise, use the exercise finder in chapter 6 or consult a professional. Remember to use a spotter in all free-weight exercises that require one (these are designated throughout chapter 6).

- Guidelines for the duration and type of warm-up and cool-down activities.
- A recommendation for the length of the *rest period* (the time you should spend recovering between sets and exercises). During this period, relax by simply sitting or standing at your exercise station, lightly stretching the muscles that you have just exercised, or preparing the bar, dumbbell, or machine for your next set or exercise.
- Workout tips that give more detail about how to complete that specific workout, answers to common questions or concerns, or suggestions about getting the most out of your training.

### Green Zone

The Green Zone is for you if you are new to weight training or if you have not been weight training recently and have a low fitness status based on the bench press test. The very low-intensity workouts in this zone initiate you gradually to weight training and make you feel more confident and comfortable in the weight room.

### Blue Zone

Blue Zone workouts are for you if you have been weight training recently on a consistent basis and have a low fitness status based on the bench press test, or if you completed Green Zone workouts and are looking for a more advanced program. The workouts in this zone provide a solid base for the more intense zones to follow.

### Purple Zone

Purple Zone workouts are for you if you have not been weight training recently on a consistent basis and have an average fitness status based on the bench press test, or if you completed Blue Zone workouts and are looking for a more advanced program. The workouts in this zone are more intense, and they help provide a base for the workouts in the advanced zones.

### Yellow Zone

Yellow Zone workouts are for you if you have been weight training recently on a consistent basis and have an average fitness status based on the bench press test, or if you completed Purple Zone workouts and are looking for a more advanced program. The workouts in this zone will help you prepare for more intense workouts of the last two zones.

### Orange Zone

Orange Zone workouts are for you if have not been weight training recently on a consistent basis and have a high fitness status based on the bench press test, or if you completed Yellow Zone workouts and are looking for a more advanced program. The workouts in this zone are intense and require dedication if you want to be successful.

### Red Zone

Red Zone workouts are for you if you have been weight training recently on a consistent basis and have a high fitness status based on the bench press test, or if you completed Orange Zone workouts and are looking for a more advanced program. The workouts in this zone represent a serious commitment to following an advanced program.

## Note About the Purple-Red Zones

Although an average or high score from the bench press test is good, realize that the Purple-Red Zones are challenging to everyone, especially if you have not been weight training recently on a consistent basis. If you feel that the workouts in your starting zone are too difficult, move to an easier one.

After you have completed the workouts in each zone, you have the option to repeat the zone, continue to the next zone, or design your own personalized program. If you are curious about your progress, you can reassess yourself in the bench press test described in chapter 3. Whatever path you choose, be sure to follow the guidelines in chapter 13 to ensure your continued success. Good luck!

# Green Zone

# 7

The Green Zone is for you if you are new to weight training or if you have not been weight training recently and have a low fitness classification in chapter 3. The very low-intensity workouts in this zone gradually initiate you to weight training and to make you feel more confident and comfortable in the weight room.

## Zone Highlights

The Green Zone covers three two-week workouts for each training outcome. There is one exercise—called a *foundational exercise* in the other color zones—for each of the seven major muscle groups: chest, back, shoulders, front of upper arm (biceps), back of upper arm (triceps), thighs, and core.

If you do not have the necessary equipment or you do not feel comfortable or experienced enough to perform any of the three exercises listed for a muscle group, go to the exercise finder in chapter 6 to choose a replacement exercise for the same muscle group. Further, if you want some variety at any point in your program, you can also find a replacement exercise as long as it trains the same muscle group. Be aware, though, that your strength will not be the same because you are not used to performing the new exercise.

### Muscle Toning

- The muscle toning program begins with two workouts a week that consist of one set of 12 to 15 repetitions for seven exercises.
- The number of sets increases from one to two in the third week, and by the fifth week you will be performing those two sets back to back.

### Body Shaping

- The body shaping program begins with three workouts per week that consist of one set of 12 to 15 repetitions for seven exercises.
- The number of sets increases from one to two in the third week, and by the fifth week you will be performing those two sets back to back.

### Strength Training

- The strength training program begins with three workouts per week that consist of one set of 12 to 15 repetitions for seven exercises.
- The number of sets increases from one to two in the third week, and by the fifth week you will be performing those two sets back to back.

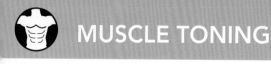

## WORKOUT 1

**Total time:**           44 minutes

**Weeks:**                1 and 2

**Days of the week:**   Two nonconsecutive days*

**Warm-up:**          Easy jogging or rope skipping for 5 minutes followed by stretching

**Exercises:**         14 minutes

|  |  |  |  | Choose 1 exercise per row | | |
| # | Muscle group | Reps | Sets | Barbell | Machine | Alternative |
|---|---|---|---|---|---|---|
| 1 | Chest | 12-15 | 1 | Bench press | Chest press | Bench press (DB) |
| 2 | Back | 12-15 | 1 | Bent-over row | Seated row | One-arm row (DB) |
| 3 | Shoulders | 12-15 | 1 | Standing press | Shoulder press | Lateral raise (DB) |
| 4 | Front of arm | 12-15 | 1 | Biceps curl | Low pulley curl | Biceps curl (DB) |
| 5 | Back of arm | 12-15 | 1 | Lying triceps extension | Triceps pushdown | Triceps kickback (DB) |
| 6 | Thighs | 12-15 | 1 | Lunge | Leg press | Squat (DB) |
| 7 | Core | 12-15 | 1 | Good morning | Abdominal crunch | Sit-up (BW) |

**Rest period:**      30 seconds**

**Cool-down:**      Slow walking for 5 minutes followed by stretching

**Workout tips:**   * Spread out your weight training sessions throughout the week; you need at least one rest day (but no more than three) between workouts. A common two-day-per-week program is Monday and Thursday or Wednesday and one weekend day.

** You may want to rest for up to 60 seconds between exercises for your first or second week of training, or both.

GREEN ZONE

## WORKOUT 2

| | |
|---|---|
| **Total time:** | 51 minutes |
| **Weeks:** | 3 and 4 |
| **Days of the week:** | Two nonconsecutive days |
| **Warm-up:** | Easy jogging or rope skipping for 5 minutes followed by stretching |
| **Exercises:** | 21 minutes |

|  |  |  |  | Choose 1 exercise per row | | |
|---|---|---|---|---|---|---|
| # | Muscle group | Reps | Sets* | Barbell | Machine | Alternative |
| 1 | Chest | 12-15 | 2 | Bench press | Chest press | Bench press (DB) |
| 2 | Back | 12-15 | 2 | Bent-over row | Seated row | One-arm row (DB) |
| 3 | Shoulders | 12-15 | 2 | Standing press | Shoulder press | Lateral raise (DB) |
| 4 | Front of arm | 12-15 | 2 | Biceps curl | Low-pulley curl | Biceps curl (DB) |
| 5 | Back of arm | 12-15 | 2 | Lying triceps extension | Triceps pushdown | Triceps kickback (DB) |
| 6 | Thighs | 12-15 | 2 | Lunge | Leg press | Squat (DB) |
| 7 | Core | 12-15 | 2 | Good morning | Abdominal crunch | Sit-up (BW) |

| | |
|---|---|
| **Rest period:** | 30 seconds |
| **Cool-down:** | Slow walking for 5 minutes followed by stretching |
| **Workout tips:** | * Complete one set of each exercise and then start over and perform the second set of each exercise (as opposed to doing two sets of each exercise back to back). |

GREEN ZONE

## WORKOUT 3

| | |
|---|---|
| **Total time:** | 51 minutes |
| **Weeks:** | 5 and 6 |
| **Days of the week:** | Two nonconsecutive days |
| **Warm-up:** | Easy jogging or rope skipping for 5 minutes followed by stretching |
| **Exercises:** | 21 minutes |

Choose 1 exercise per row

| # | Muscle group | Reps | Sets* | Barbell | Machine | Alternative |
|---|---|---|---|---|---|---|
| 1 | Chest | 12-15 | 2 | Bench press | Chest press | Bench press (DB) |
| 2 | Back | 12-15 | 2 | Bent-over row | Seated row | One-arm row (DB) |
| 3 | Shoulders | 12-15 | 2 | Standing press | Shoulder press | Lateral raise (DB) |
| 4 | Front of arm | 12-15 | 2 | Biceps curl | Low-pulley curl | Biceps curl (DB) |
| 5 | Back of arm | 12-15 | 2 | Lying triceps extension | Triceps pushdown | Triceps kickback (DB) |
| 6 | Thighs | 12-15 | 2 | Lunge | Leg press | Squat (DB) |
| 7 | Core | 12-15 | 2 | Good morning | Abdominal crunch | Sit-up (BW) |

| | |
|---|---|
| **Rest period:** | 30 seconds |
| **Cool-down:** | Slow walking for 5 minutes followed by stretching |
| **Workout tip:** | * At this point you should be able to perform the required two sets back to back. |

## WORKOUT 1

| | |
|---|---|
| **Total time:** | 44 minutes |
| **Weeks:** | 1 and 2 |
| **Days of the week:** | Three nonconsecutive days* |
| **Warm-up:** | Easy jogging or rope skipping for 5 minutes followed by stretching |
| **Exercises:** | 14 minutes |

| | | | | Choose 1 exercise per row | | |
|---|---|---|---|---|---|---|
| # | Muscle group | Reps | Sets | Barbell | Machine | Alternative |
| 1 | Chest | 12-15 | 1 | Bench press | Chest press | Bench press (DB) |
| 2 | Back | 12-15 | 1 | Bent-over row | Seated row | One-arm row (DB) |
| 3 | Shoulders | 12-15 | 1 | Standing press | Shoulder press | Lateral raise (DB) |
| 4 | Front of arm | 12-15 | 1 | Biceps curl | Low-pulley curl | Biceps curl (DB) |
| 5 | Back of arm | 12-15 | 1 | Lying triceps extension | Triceps pushdown | Triceps kickback (DB) |
| 6 | Thighs | 12-15 | 1 | Lunge | Leg press | Squat (DB) |
| 7 | Core | 12-15 | 1 | Good morning | Abdominal crunch | Sit-up (BW) |

| | |
|---|---|
| **Rest period:** | 30 seconds** |
| **Cool-down:** | Slow walking for 5 minutes followed by stretching |
| **Workout tips:** | * Spread out your weight training sessions throughout the week; you need at least one rest day (but no more than three) between workouts. A common three-day-per-week program is Monday, Wednesday, and Friday or Tuesday, Thursday, and one weekend day. |
| | ** You may want to rest for up to 60 seconds between exercises for your first or second week of training, or both. |

GREEN ZONE

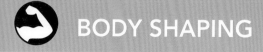

## WORKOUT 2

| | |
|---|---|
| **Total time:** | 51 minutes |
| **Weeks:** | 3 and 4 |
| **Days of the week:** | Three nonconsecutive days |
| **Warm-up:** | Easy jogging or rope skipping for 5 minutes followed by stretching |
| **Exercises:** | 21 minutes |

| | | | | Choose 1 exercise per row | | |
|---|---|---|---|---|---|---|
| # | Muscle group | Reps | Sets* | Barbell | Machine | Alternative |
| 1 | Chest | 12-15 | 2 | Bench press | Chest press | Bench press (DB) |
| 2 | Back | 12-15 | 2 | Bent-over row | Seated row | One-arm row (DB) |
| 3 | Shoulders | 12-15 | 2 | Standing press | Shoulder press | Lateral raise (DB) |
| 4 | Front of arm | 12-15 | 2 | Biceps curl | Low-pulley curl | Biceps curl (DB) |
| 5 | Back of arm | 12-15 | 2 | Lying triceps extension | Triceps pushdown | Triceps kickback (DB) |
| 6 | Thighs | 12-15 | 2 | Lunge | Leg press | Squat (DB) |
| 7 | Core | 12-15 | 2 | Good morning | Abdominal crunch | Sit-up (BW) |

| | |
|---|---|
| **Rest period:** | 30 seconds |
| **Cool-down:** | Slow walking for 5 minutes followed by stretching |
| **Workout tips:** | * Complete one set of each exercise and then start over and perform the second set of each exercise (as opposed to doing two sets of each exercise back to back). |

## WORKOUT 3

| | |
|---|---|
| **Total time:** | 51 minutes |
| **Weeks:** | 5 and 6 |
| **Days of the week:** | Three nonconsecutive days |
| **Warm-up:** | Easy jogging or rope skipping for 5 minutes followed by stretching |
| **Exercises:** | 21 minutes |

| | | | | Choose 1 exercise per row | | |
|---|---|---|---|---|---|---|
| **#** | **Muscle group** | **Reps** | **Sets*** | **Barbell** | **Machine** | **Alternative** |
| 1 | Chest | 12-15 | 2 | Bench press | Chest press | Bench press (DB) |
| 2 | Back | 12-15 | 2 | Bent-over row | Seated row | One-arm row (DB) |
| 3 | Shoulders | 12-15 | 2 | Standing press | Shoulder press | Lateral raise (DB) |
| 4 | Front of arm | 12-15 | 2 | Biceps curl | Low-pulley curl | Biceps curl (DB) |
| 5 | Back of arm | 12-15 | 2 | Lying triceps extension | Triceps pushdown | Triceps kickback (DB) |
| 6 | Thighs | 12-15 | 2 | Lunge | Leg press | Squat (DB) |
| 7 | Core | 12-15 | 2 | Good morning | Abdominal crunch | Sit-up (BW) |

| | |
|---|---|
| **Rest period:** | 30 seconds |
| **Cool-down:** | Slow walking for 5 minutes followed by stretching |
| **Workout tips:** | * At this point you should be able to perform the required two sets back to back. |

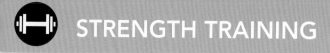
## WORKOUT 1

| | |
|---|---|
| **Total time:** | 44 minutes |
| **Weeks:** | 1 and 2 |
| **Days of the week:** | Three nonconsecutive days* |
| **Warm-up:** | Easy jogging or rope skipping for 5 minutes followed by stretching |
| **Exercises:** | 14 minutes |

| | | | | Choose 1 exercise per row | | |
|---|---|---|---|---|---|---|
| **#** | **Muscle group** | **Reps** | **Sets** | **Barbell** | **Machine** | **Alternative** |
| 1 | Chest | 12-15 | 1 | Bench press | Chest press | Bench press (DB) |
| 2 | Back | 12-15 | 1 | Bent-over row | Seated row | One-arm row (DB) |
| 3 | Shoulders | 12-15 | 1 | Standing press | Shoulder press | Lateral raise (DB) |
| 4 | Front of arm | 12-15 | 1 | Biceps curl | Low-pulley curl | Biceps curl (DB) |
| 5 | Back of arm | 12-15 | 1 | Lying triceps extension | Triceps pushdown | Triceps kickback (DB) |
| 6 | Thighs | 12-15 | 1 | Lunge | Leg press | Squat (DB) |
| 7 | Core | 12-15 | 1 | Good morning | Abdominal crunch | Sit-up (BW) |

| | |
|---|---|
| **Rest period:** | 30 seconds** |
| **Cool-down:** | Slow walking for 5 minutes followed by stretching |
| **Workout tips:** | * Spread out your weight training sessions throughout the week; you need at least one rest day (but no more than three) between workouts. A common three-day-per-week program is Monday, Wednesday, and Friday or Tuesday, Thursday, and one weekend day. |
| | ** You may want to rest for up to 60 seconds between exercises for your first or second week of training, or both. |

GREEN ZONE

## WORKOUT 2

| | |
|---|---|
| **Total time:** | 51 minutes |
| **Weeks:** | 3 and 4 |
| **Days of the week:** | Three nonconsecutive days |
| **Warm-up:** | Easy jogging or rope skipping for 5 minutes followed by stretching |
| **Exercises:** | 21 minutes |

| | | | | Choose 1 exercise per row | | |
|---|---|---|---|---|---|---|
| # | Muscle group | Reps | Sets* | Barbell | Machine | Alternative |
| 1 | Chest | 12-15 | 2 | Bench press | Chest press | Bench press (DB) |
| 2 | Back | 12-15 | 2 | Bent-over row | Seated row | One-arm row (DB) |
| 3 | Shoulders | 12-15 | 2 | Standing press | Shoulder press | Lateral raise (DB) |
| 4 | Front of arm | 12-15 | 2 | Biceps curl | Low-pulley curl | Biceps curl (DB) |
| 5 | Back of arm | 12-15 | 2 | Lying triceps extension | Triceps pushdown | Triceps kickback (DB) |
| 6 | Thighs | 12-15 | 2 | Lunge | Leg press | Squat (DB) |
| 7 | Core | 12-15 | 2 | Good morning | Abdominal crunch | Sit-up (BW) |

| | |
|---|---|
| **Rest period:** | 30 seconds |
| **Cool-down:** | Slow walking for 5 minutes followed by stretching |
| **Workout tips:** | * Complete one set of each exercise and then start over and perform the second set of each exercise (as opposed to doing two sets of each exercise back to back). |

## WORKOUT 3

| | |
|---|---|
| **Total time:** | 51 minutes |
| **Weeks:** | 5 and 6 |
| **Days of the week:** | Three nonconsecutive days |
| **Warm-up:** | Easy jogging or rope skipping for 5 minutes followed by stretching |
| **Exercises:** | 21 minutes |

| | | | | Choose 1 exercise per row | | |
|---|---|---|---|---|---|---|
| # | Muscle group | Reps | Sets* | Barbell | Machine | Alternative |
| 1 | Chest | 12-15 | 2 | Bench press | Chest press | Bench press (DB) |
| 2 | Back | 12-15 | 2 | Bent-over row | Seated row | One-arm row (DB) |
| 3 | Shoulders | 12-15 | 2 | Standing press | Shoulder press | Lateral raise (DB) |
| 4 | Front of arm | 12-15 | 2 | Biceps curl | Low-pulley curl | Biceps curl (DB) |
| 5 | Back of arm | 12-15 | 2 | Lying triceps extension | Triceps pushdown | Triceps kickback (DB) |
| 6 | Thighs | 12-15 | 2 | Lunge | Leg press | Squat (DB) |
| 7 | Core | 12-15 | 2 | Good morning | Abdominal crunch | Sit-up (BW) |

| | |
|---|---|
| **Rest period:** | 30 seconds |
| **Cool-down:** | Slow walking for 5 minutes followed by stretching |
| **Workout tips:** | * At this point you should be able to perform the required two sets back to back. |

# 8

# Blue Zone

The Blue Zone is for you if you have been weight training recently on a consistent basis but scored in the low fitness classification in chapter 3, or if you completed the Green Zone and are looking for a more advanced program. The workouts in this zone provide a solid base for the more intense zones to follow.

## Zone Highlights

The Blue Zone covers three two-week workouts for each training outcome. The foundational exercises include one exercise for each of the seven major muscle groups: chest, back, shoulders, front of upper arm (biceps), back of upper arm (triceps), thighs, and core.

If you do not have the necessary equipment or you do not feel comfortable or experienced enough to perform any of the three exercises listed for a muscle group, go to the exercise finder in chapter 6 to choose a replacement exercise for the same muscle group. Further, if you want some variety at any point in your program, you can also find a replacement exercise as long as it trains the same muscle group. Be aware, though, that your strength will not be the same because you are not used to performing the new exercise. Use the guidelines in chapter 4 to determine your starting load and then adjust that load using tables 4.10 or 4.11 to match the number of repetitions (e.g., 10-12 rather than 12-15) that is listed in your zone workout table for that muscle group.

### Muscle Toning

The muscle toning program continues the 12 to 15 repetitions from the Green Zone and gradually adds another set. (By the fifth week you will be doing three back-to-back sets.)

### Body Shaping

The body shaping program gradually decreases the number of repetitions to 10 to 12 but retains three sessions a week. Remember, as the number of repetitions decreases, you should increase the loads (chapter 4 can assist you in this process).

## Strength Training

- Weeks 1 and 2 decrease the number of repetitions to 10 to 12 in the second set (only) of all exercises. Be sure to increase the weight slightly in the second set (see chapter 4).
- Weeks 3 and 4 require that you perform both sets with a slightly heavier weight for 10 to 12 repetitions in all exercises.
- Weeks 5 and 6 again decrease the number of repetitions (which means that you need to add weight) to 8 to 10 in the second set (only) of the three major exercises (those that train the chest, shoulders, and thighs).

## WORKOUT 1

| | |
|---|---|
| **Total time:** | 56 minutes |
| **Weeks:** | 1 and 2 |
| **Days of the week:** | Two nonconsecutive days |
| **Warm-up:** | Easy jogging or rope skipping for 5 minutes followed by stretching |
| **Exercises:** | 26 minutes |

| | | | | Choose 1 exercise per row | | |
|---|---|---|---|---|---|---|
| **#** | **Muscle group** | **Reps** | **Sets*** | **Barbell** | **Machine** | **Alternative** |
| 1 | Chest | 12-15 | 3** | Bench press | Chest press | Bench press (DB) |
| 2 | Back | 12-15 | 2 | Bent-over row | Seated row | One-arm row (DB) |
| 3 | Shoulders | 12-15 | 3** | Standing press | Shoulder press | Lateral raise (DB) |
| 4 | Front of arm | 12-15 | 2 | Biceps curl | Low-pulley curl | Biceps curl (DB) |
| 5 | Back of arm | 12-15 | 2 | Lying triceps extension | Triceps pushdown | Triceps kickback (DB) |
| 6 | Thighs | 12-15 | 3** | Lunge | Leg press | Squat (DB) |
| 7 | Core | 12-15 | 2 | Good morning | Abdominal crunch | Sit-up (BW) |

| | |
|---|---|
| **Rest period:** | 30 seconds |
| **Cool-down:** | Slow walking for 5 minutes followed by stretching |
| **Workout tips:** | * Do two sets of each exercise back to back. |
| | ** After doing two sets of all exercises, come back and perform the last (third) set of exercises 1, 3, and 6 in this order: 1, 6, and then 3. |

BLUE ZONE

## WORKOUT 2

| | |
|---|---|
| **Total time:** | 56 minutes |
| **Weeks:** | 3 and 4 |
| **Days of the week:** | Two nonconsecutive days |
| **Warm-up:** | Easy jogging or rope skipping for 5 minutes followed by stretching |
| **Exercises:** | 26 minutes |

| | | | | Choose 1 exercise per row | | |
|---|---|---|---|---|---|---|
| **#** | **Muscle group** | **Reps** | **Sets*** | **Barbell** | **Machine** | **Alternative** |
| 1 | Chest | 12-15 | 3 | Bench press | Chest press | Bench press (DB) |
| 2 | Back | 12-15 | 2 | Bent-over row | Seated row | One-arm row (DB) |
| 3 | Shoulders | 12-15 | 3 | Standing press | Shoulder press | Lateral raise (DB) |
| 4 | Front of arm | 12-15 | 2 | Biceps curl | Low-pulley curl | Biceps curl (DB) |
| 5 | Back of arm | 12-15 | 2 | Lying triceps extension | Triceps pushdown | Triceps kickback (DB) |
| 6 | Thighs | 12-15 | 3 | Lunge | Leg press | Squat (DB) |
| 7 | Core | 12-15 | 2 | Good morning | Abdominal crunch | Sit-up (BW) |

| | |
|---|---|
| **Rest period:** | 30 seconds |
| **Cool-down:** | Slow walking for 5 minutes followed by stretching |
| **Workout tips:** | * At this point you should be able to perform the required two or three sets back to back. |

## WORKOUT 3

| | |
|---|---|
| **Total time:** | 1 hour, 2 minutes |
| **Weeks:** | 5 and 6 |
| **Days of the week:** | Two nonconsecutive days |
| **Warm-up:** | Easy jogging or rope skipping for 5 minutes followed by stretching |
| **Exercises:** | 32 minutes |

| | | | | Choose 1 exercise per row | | |
|---|---|---|---|---|---|---|
| **#** | **Muscle group** | **Reps** | **Sets\*** | **Barbell** | **Machine** | **Alternative** |
| 1 | Chest | 12-15 | 3 | Bench press | Chest press | Bench press (DB) |
| 2 | Back | 12-15 | 3 | Bent-over row | Seated row | One-arm row (DB) |
| 3 | Shoulders | 12-15 | 3 | Standing press | Shoulder press | Lateral raise (DB) |
| 4 | Front of arm | 12-15 | 3 | Biceps curl | Low-pulley curl | Biceps curl (DB) |
| 5 | Back of arm | 12-15 | 3 | Lying triceps extension | Triceps pushdown | Triceps kickback (DB) |
| 6 | Thighs | 12-15 | 3 | Lunge | Leg press | Squat (DB) |
| 7 | Core | 12-15 | 3 | Good morning | Abdominal crunch | Sit-up (BW) |

| | |
|---|---|
| **Rest period:** | 30 seconds |
| **Cool-down:** | Slow walking for 5 minutes followed by stretching |
| **Workout tips:** | \* At this point you should be able to perform the required three sets back to back. |

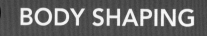
## WORKOUT 1

| | |
|---|---|
| **Total time:** | 52 minutes |
| **Weeks:** | 1 and 2 |
| **Days of the week:** | Three nonconsecutive days |
| **Warm-up:** | Easy jogging or rope skipping for 5 minutes followed by stretching |
| **Exercises:** | 22 minutes |

| | | | | Choose 1 exercise per row | | |
|---|---|---|---|---|---|---|
| **#** | **Muscle group** | **Reps** | **Sets** | **Barbell** | **Machine** | **Alternative** |
| 1 | Chest | 12-15<br>10-12* | 1<br>1 | Bench press | Chest press | Bench press (DB) |
| 2 | Back | 12-15 | 2 | Bent-over row | Seated row | One-arm row (DB) |
| 3 | Shoulders | 12-15<br>10-12* | 1<br>1 | Standing press | Shoulder press | Lateral raise (DB) |
| 4 | Front of arm | 12-15 | 2 | Biceps curl | Low-pulley curl | Biceps curl (DB) |
| 5 | Back of arm | 12-15 | 2 | Lying triceps extension | Triceps pushdown | Triceps kickback (DB) |
| 6 | Thighs | 12-15<br>10-12* | 1<br>1 | Lunge | Leg press | Squat (DB) |
| 7 | Core | 15-25** | 2 | Good morning | Abdominal crunch | Sit-up (BW) |

| | |
|---|---|
| **Rest period:** | 60 seconds after sets of 10 to 12 repetitions***; 30 seconds after sets of 12 to 15 repetitions |
| **Cool-down:** | Slow walking for 5 minutes followed by stretching |
| **Workout tips:** | * When you make the change to performing sets of 10 to 12 repetitions instead of 12 to 15 repetitions, a general guideline is to add 5 to 10 pounds (~2.5-5 kg) to your upper-body exercises and 10 to 20 pounds (~5-10 kg) to your lower-body exercises. At this point you have to lift only the heavier weight (and perform fewer repetitions) in the second of the two sets for exercises 1, 3, and 6. |
| | ** You are now doing sets of 15 to 25 repetitions for your core exercise. |
| | *** The rest period after these heavier sets is longer (60 seconds versus 30 seconds). |

## WORKOUT 2

**Total time:**          53 minutes

**Weeks:**               3 and 4

**Days of the week:**    Three nonconsecutive days

**Warm-up:**             Easy jogging or rope skipping for 5 minutes followed by stretching

**Exercises:**           23 minutes

|  |  |  |  | Choose 1 exercise per row | | |
|---|---|---|---|---|---|---|
| # | Muscle group | Reps | Sets | Barbell | Machine | Alternative |
| 1 | Chest | 10-12 | 2* | Bench press | Chest press | Bench press (DB) |
| 2 | Back | 12-15 | 2 | Bent-over row | Seated row | One-arm row (DB) |
| 3 | Shoulders | 10-12 | 2* | Standing press | Shoulder press | Lateral raise (DB) |
| 4 | Front of arm | 12-15 | 2 | Biceps curl | Low-pulley curl | Biceps curl (DB) |
| 5 | Back of arm | 12-15 | 2 | Lying triceps extension | Triceps pushdown | Triceps kickback (DB) |
| 6 | Thighs | 10-12 | 2* | Lunge | Leg press | Squat (DB) |
| 7 | Core | 15-25 | 2 | Good morning | Abdominal crunch | Sit-up (BW) |

**Rest period:**     60 seconds for exercises 1, 3, and 6; 30 seconds for exercises 2, 4, 5, and 7

**Cool-down:**      Slow walking for 5 minutes followed by stretching

**Workout tips:**   * As you begin performing both sets with the heavier load (for fewer repetitions) for exercises 1, 3, and 6, you may have to decrease the load slightly in the second set to complete both sets successfully.

BLUE ZONE

## WORKOUT 3

| | |
|---|---|
| **Total time:** | 55 minutes |
| **Weeks:** | 5 and 6 |
| **Days of the week:** | Three nonconsecutive days |
| **Warm-up:** | Easy jogging or rope skipping for 5 minutes followed by stretching |
| **Exercises:** | 25 minutes |

| | | | | Choose 1 exercise per row | | |
|---|---|---|---|---|---|---|
| **#** | **Muscle group** | **Reps** | **Sets** | **Barbell** | **Machine** | **Alternative** |
| 1 | Chest | 10-12 | 2 | Bench press | Chest press | Bench press (DB) |
| 2 | Back | 10-12* | 2** | Bent-over row | Seated row | One-arm row (DB) |
| 3 | Shoulders | 10-12 | 2 | Standing press | Shoulder press | Lateral raise (DB) |
| 4 | Front of arm | 10-12* | 2** | Biceps curl | Low-pulley curl | Biceps curl (DB) |
| 5 | Back of arm | 10-12* | 2** | Lying triceps extension | Triceps pushdown | Triceps kickback (DB) |
| 6 | Thighs | 10-12 | 2 | Lunge | Leg press | Squat (DB) |
| 7 | Core | 15-25 | 2 | Good morning | Abdominal crunch | Sit-up (BW) |

| | |
|---|---|
| **Rest period:** | 1 minute |
| **Cool-down:** | Slow walking for 5 minutes followed by stretching |
| **Workout tips:** | * When you make the change to performing sets of 10 to 12 repetitions instead of 12 to 15 repetitions for upper-body exercises 2, 4, and 5, a general guideline is to add 5 to 10 pounds (~2.5-5 kg). |
| | ** As you begin performing both sets with the heavier load (for fewer repetitions), you may have to decrease the load slightly in the second set to complete both sets successfully. |

## WORKOUT 1

| | | |
|---|---|---|
| **Total time:** | 53 minutes |
| **Weeks:** | 1 and 2 |
| **Days of the week:** | Three nonconsecutive days |
| **Warm-up:** | Easy jogging or rope skipping for 5 minutes followed by stretching |
| **Exercises:** | 23 minutes |

| | | | | Choose 1 exercise per row | | |
|---|---|---|---|---|---|---|
| **#** | **Muscle group** | **Reps** | **Sets** | **Barbell** | **Machine** | **Alternative** |
| 1 | Chest | 12-15<br>10-12* | 1<br>1 | Bench press | Chest press | Bench press (DB) |
| 2 | Back | 12-15<br>10-12* | 1<br>1 | Bent-over row | Seated row | One-arm row (DB) |
| 3 | Shoulders | 12-15<br>10-12* | 1<br>1 | Standing press | Shoulder press | Lateral raise (DB) |
| 4 | Front of arm | 12-15<br>10-12* | 1<br>1 | Biceps curl | Low-pulley curl | Biceps curl (DB) |
| 5 | Back of arm | 12-15<br>10-12* | 1<br>1 | Lying triceps extension | Triceps pushdown | Triceps kickback (DB) |
| 6 | Thighs | 12-15<br>10-12* | 1<br>1 | Lunge | Leg press | Squat (DB) |
| 7 | Core | 15-25** | 2 | Good morning | Abdominal crunch | Sit-up (BW) |

| | |
|---|---|
| **Rest period:** | 1 minute after sets of 10 to 12 repetitions***; 30 seconds after sets of 12 to 15 repetitions |
| **Cool-down:** | Slow walking for 5 minutes followed by stretching |
| **Workout tips:** | * When you make the change to performing sets of 10 to 12 repetitions instead of 12 to 15 repetitions, a general guideline is to add 5 to 10 pounds (~2.5-5 kg) to your upper-body exercises and 10 to 20 pounds (~5-10 kg) to your lower-body exercises. At this point you have to lift the heavier weight (and perform fewer repetitions) only in the second of the two sets. |

** You are now doing sets of 15 to 25 repetitions for your core exercise.

*** The rest period after these heavier sets is longer (60 seconds versus 30 seconds).

## WORKOUT 2

| | |
|---|---|
| **Total time:** | 55 minutes |
| **Weeks:** | 3 and 4 |
| **Days of the week:** | Three nonconsecutive days |
| **Warm-up:** | Easy jogging or rope skipping for 5 minutes followed by stretching |
| **Exercises:** | 25 minutes |

| | | | | Choose 1 exercise per row | | |
|---|---|---|---|---|---|---|
| **#** | **Muscle group** | **Reps** | **Sets*** | **Barbell** | **Machine** | **Alternative** |
| 1 | Chest | 10-12 | 2 | Bench press | Chest press | Bench press (DB) |
| 2 | Back | 10-12 | 2 | Bent-over row | Seated row | One-arm row (DB) |
| 3 | Shoulders | 10-12 | 2 | Standing press | Shoulder press | Lateral raise (DB) |
| 4 | Front of arm | 10-12 | 2 | Biceps curl | Low-pulley curl | Biceps curl (DB) |
| 5 | Back of arm | 10-12 | 2 | Lying triceps extension | Triceps pushdown | Triceps kickback (DB) |
| 6 | Thighs | 10-12 | 2 | Lunge | Leg press | Squat (DB) |
| 7 | Core | 15-25 | 2 | Good morning | Abdominal crunch | Sit-up (BW) |

| | |
|---|---|
| **Rest period:** | 1 minute |
| **Cool-down:** | Slow walking for 5 minutes followed by stretching |
| **Workout tips:** | * As you begin performing both sets with the heavier load (for fewer repetitions), you may have to decrease the load slightly in the second set to complete both sets. |

## WORKOUT 3

| | |
|---|---|
| **Total time:** | 55 minutes |
| **Weeks:** | 5 and 6 |
| **Days of the week:** | Three nonconsecutive days |
| **Warm-up:** | Easy jogging or rope skipping for 5 minutes followed by stretching |
| **Exercises:** | 25 minutes |

| | | | | Choose 1 exercise per row | | |
|---|---|---|---|---|---|---|
| **#** | **Muscle group** | **Reps** | **Sets** | **Barbell** | **Machine** | **Alternative** |
| 1 | Chest | 10-12<br>8-10* | 1<br>1 | Bench press | Chest press | Bench press (DB) |
| 2 | Back | 10-12 | 2 | Bent-over row | Seated row | One-arm row (DB) |
| 3 | Shoulders | 10-12<br>8-10* | 1<br>1 | Standing press | Shoulder press | Lateral raise (DB) |
| 4 | Front of arm | 10-12 | 2 | Biceps curl | Low-pulley curl | Biceps curl (DB) |
| 5 | Back of arm | 10-12 | 2 | Lying triceps extension | Triceps pushdown | Triceps kickback (DB) |
| 6 | Thighs | 10-12<br>8-10* | 1<br>1 | Lunge | Leg press | Squat (DB) |
| 7 | Core | 15-25 | 2 | Good morning | Abdominal crunch | Sit-up (BW) |

| | |
|---|---|
| **Rest period:** | 1 minute |
| **Cool-down:** | Slow walking for 5 minutes followed by stretching |
| **Workout tips:** | * When you make the change to performing sets of 8 to 10 repetitions instead of 10 to 12 repetitions, a general guideline is to add 5 to 10 pounds (~2.5-5 kg) to your upper-body exercises and 10 to 20 pounds (~5-10 kg) to your lower-body exercises. At this point you have to lift the heavier weight (and perform fewer repetitions) only in the second of the two sets for exercises 1, 3, and 6. |

BLUE ZONE

# 9

# Purple Zone

The Purple Zone is for you if you have not been weight training recently on a consistent basis and scored in the average fitness classification in chapter 3, or if you completed the Blue Zone and are looking for a more advanced program. The workouts in this zone are more intense, and they help provide a base for the workouts in the advanced zones.

## Zone Highlights

The Purple Zone covers multiple two-week workouts for each training outcome. The foundational exercises include one exercise for each of the seven major muscle groups: chest, back, shoulders, front of upper arm (biceps), back of upper arm (triceps), thighs, and core. This zone adds upper-body and lower-body exercises to the strength training workouts.

If you do not have the necessary equipment or you do not feel comfortable or experienced enough to perform any of the three exercises listed for a muscle group, go to the exercise finder in chapter 6 to choose a replacement exercise for the same muscle group. Further, if you want some variety at any point in your program, you can also find a replacement exercise as long as it trains the same muscle group. Be aware, though, that your strength will not be the same because you are not used to performing the new exercise. Use the guidelines in chapter 4 to determine your starting load and then adjust that load using tables 4.10 or 4.11 to match the number of repetitions (e.g., 10-12 rather than 12-15) that is listed in your zone workout table for that muscle group.

### Muscle Toning

A major change in this zone is that you will be completing three workouts a week instead of two. Because of this increase, weeks 1 and 2 require you to complete only two sets per exercise. Weeks 3 through 6 gradually return you to two or three back-to-back sets.

## Body Shaping

The six weeks of this zone gradually train you to be able to perform 10 to 12 repetitions in three back-to-back sets for the seven original exercises.

## Strength Training

- A major change in this zone is that you will be completing four workouts each week; your program includes two upper-body and two lower-body training days. Because of the increase in the number of weekly workouts, weeks 1 and 2 will require only one set of 10 to 12 repetitions in the two new upper-body exercises and the four new lower-body exercises. (An exception is that you will do 8 to 10 repetitions in the new thigh exercise.) The upper-body exercises include two each for the chest and back and one each for the shoulders, front of upper arm (biceps), and back of upper arm (triceps). The lower-body exercises include two for the thighs and one each for the back of thigh (hamstrings), front of thigh (quadriceps), calves, and core. Chapter 4 will help you determine the loads for your new exercises.
- Weeks 3 through 6 gradually increase the number of sets so that you will be performing three back-to-back sets in the two major upper-body exercises (a chest exercise and the shoulder exercise) and in the two major lower-body exercises (both thigh exercises). The other exercises require only two sets.

## WORKOUT 1

| | |
|---|---|
| **Total time:** | 51 minutes |
| **Weeks:** | 1 and 2 |
| **Days of the week:** | Three nonconsecutive days* |
| **Warm-up:** | Easy jogging or rope skipping for 5 minutes followed by stretching |
| **Exercises:** | 21 minutes |

|   |                   |        |      | **Choose 1 exercise per row** | | |
|---|-------------------|--------|------|---------------------|------------------|------------------------|
| **#** | **Muscle group** | **Reps** | **Sets** | **Barbell** | **Machine** | **Alternative** |
| 1 | Chest | 12-15 | 2 | Bench press | Chest press | Bench press (DB) |
| 2 | Back | 12-15 | 2 | Bent-over row | Seated row | One-arm row (DB) |
| 3 | Shoulders | 12-15 | 2 | Standing press | Shoulder press | Lateral raise (DB) |
| 4 | Front of arm | 12-15 | 2 | Biceps curl | Low-pulley curl | Biceps curl (DB) |
| 5 | Back of arm | 12-15 | 2 | Lying triceps extension | Triceps pushdown | Triceps kickback (DB) |
| 6 | Thighs | 12-15 | 2 | Lunge | Leg press | Squat (DB) |
| 7 | Core | 15-25** | 2 | Good morning | Abdominal crunch | Sit-up (BW) |

| | |
|---|---|
| **Rest period:** | 30 seconds |
| **Cool-down:** | Slow walking for 5 minutes followed by stretching |
| **Workout tips:** | * Spread out your weight training sessions throughout the week; you need at least one rest day (but no more than three) between workouts. A common three-day-per-week program is Monday, Wednesday, and Friday or Tuesday, Thursday, and one weekend day. |
| | ** Note that you are now doing sets of 15 to 25 repetitions for your core exercise. |

## WORKOUT 2

| | |
|---|---|
| **Total time:** | 56 minutes |
| **Weeks:** | 3 and 4 |
| **Days of the week:** | Three nonconsecutive days |
| **Warm-up:** | Easy jogging or rope skipping for 5 minutes followed by stretching |
| **Exercises:** | 26 minutes |

| | | | | Choose 1 exercise per row | | |
|---|---|---|---|---|---|---|
| **#** | **Muscle group** | **Reps** | **Sets\*** | **Barbell** | **Machine** | **Alternative** |
| 1 | Chest | 12-15 | 3** | Bench press | Chest press | Bench press (DB) |
| 2 | Back | 12-15 | 2 | Bent-over row | Seated row | One-arm row (DB) |
| 3 | Shoulders | 12-15 | 3** | Standing press | Shoulder press | Lateral raise (DB) |
| 4 | Front of arm | 12-15 | 2 | Biceps curl | Low-pulley curl | Biceps curl (DB) |
| 5 | Back of arm | 12-15 | 2 | Lying triceps extension | Triceps pushdown | Triceps kickback (DB) |
| 6 | Thighs | 12-15 | 3** | Lunge | Leg press | Squat (DB) |
| 7 | Core | 15-25 | 2 | Good morning | Abdominal crunch | Sit-up (BW) |

| | |
|---|---|
| **Rest period:** | 30 seconds |
| **Cool-down:** | Slow walking for 5 minutes followed by stretching |
| **Workout tips:** | * Do two sets of each exercise back to back. |
| | ** After doing two sets of all exercises, come back and perform the last (third) set of exercises 1, 3, and 6 in this order: 1, 6, and then 3. |

## WORKOUT 3

| | |
|---|---|
| **Total time:** | 56 minutes |
| **Weeks:** | 5 and 6 |
| **Days of the week:** | Three nonconsecutive days |
| **Warm-up:** | Easy jogging or rope skipping for 5 minutes followed by stretching |
| **Exercises:** | 26 minutes |

|  |  |  |  | Choose 1 exercise per row | | |
|---|---|---|---|---|---|---|
| **#** | **Muscle group** | **Reps** | **Sets*** | **Barbell** | **Machine** | **Alternative** |
| 1 | Chest | 12-15 | 3 | Bench press | Chest press | Bench press (DB) |
| 2 | Back | 12-15 | 2 | Bent-over row | Seated row | One-arm row (DB) |
| 3 | Shoulders | 12-15 | 3 | Standing press | Shoulder press | Lateral raise (DB) |
| 4 | Front of arm | 12-15 | 2 | Biceps curl | Low-pulley curl | Biceps curl (DB) |
| 5 | Back of arm | 12-15 | 2 | Lying triceps extension | Triceps pushdown | Triceps kickback (DB) |
| 6 | Thighs | 12-15 | 3 | Lunge | Leg press | Squat (DB) |
| 7 | Core | 15-25 | 2 | Good morning | Abdominal crunch | Sit-up (BW) |

| | |
|---|---|
| **Rest period:** | 30 seconds |
| **Cool-down:** | Slow walking for 5 minutes followed by stretching |
| **Workout tips:** | * At this point you should be able to perform the required two or three sets back to back. |

### WORKOUT 1

| | |
|---|---|
| **Total time:** | 1 hour, 1 minute |
| **Weeks:** | 1 and 2 |
| **Days of the week:** | Three nonconsecutive days |
| **Warm-up:** | Easy jogging or rope skipping for 5 minutes followed by stretching |
| **Exercises:** | 31 minutes |

| | | | | Choose 1 exercise per row | | |
|---|---|---|---|---|---|---|
| **#** | **Muscle group** | **Reps** | **Sets** | **Barbell** | **Machine** | **Alternative** |
| 1 | Chest | 10-12 | 3* | Bench press | Chest press | Bench press (DB) |
| 2 | Back | 10-12 | 2 | Bent-over row | Seated row | One-arm row (DB) |
| 3 | Shoulders | 10-12 | 3* | Standing press | Shoulder press | Lateral raise (DB) |
| 4 | Front of arm | 10-12 | 2 | Biceps curl | Low-pulley curl | Biceps curl (DB) |
| 5 | Back of arm | 10-12 | 2 | Lying triceps extension | Triceps pushdown | Triceps kickback (DB) |
| 6 | Thighs | 10-12 | 3* | Lunge | Leg press | Squat (DB) |
| 7 | Core | 15-25 | 2 | Good morning | Abdominal crunch | Sit-up (BW) |

| | |
|---|---|
| **Rest period:** | 1 minute |
| **Cool-down:** | Slow walking for 5 minutes followed by stretching |
| **Workout tips:** | * Do two sets of each exercise back to back and then come back and perform the last (third) set of exercises 1, 3, and 6 in this order: 1, 6, and then 3. |

## WORKOUT 2

| | |
|---|---|
| **Total time:** | 1 hour, 1 minute |
| **Weeks:** | 3 and 4 |
| **Days of the week:** | Three nonconsecutive days |
| **Warm-up:** | Easy jogging or rope skipping for 5 minutes followed by stretching |
| **Exercises:** | 31 minutes |

| | | | | Choose 1 exercise per row | | |
|---|---|---|---|---|---|---|
| **#** | **Muscle group** | **Reps** | **Sets*** | **Barbell** | **Machine** | **Alternative** |
| 1 | Chest | 10-12 | 3 | Bench press | Chest press | Bench press (DB) |
| 2 | Back | 10-12 | 2 | Bent-over row | Seated row | One-arm row (DB) |
| 3 | Shoulders | 10-12 | 3 | Standing press | Shoulder press | Lateral raise (DB) |
| 4 | Front of arm | 10-12 | 2 | Biceps curl | Low-pulley curl | Biceps curl (DB) |
| 5 | Back of arm | 10-12 | 2 | Lying triceps extension | Triceps pushdown | Triceps kickback (DB) |
| 6 | Thighs | 10-12 | 3 | Lunge | Leg press | Squat (DB) |
| 7 | Core | 15-25 | 2 | Good morning | Abdominal crunch | Sit-up (BW) |

| | |
|---|---|
| **Rest period:** | 1 minute |
| **Cool-down:** | Slow walking for 5 minutes followed by stretching |
| **Workout tips:** | * At this point you should be able to perform the required two or three sets back to back. |

## WORKOUT 3

| | |
|---|---|
| **Total time:** | 1 hour, 8 minutes |
| **Weeks:** | 5 and 6 |
| **Days of the week:** | Three nonconsecutive days |
| **Warm-up:** | Easy jogging or rope skipping for 5 minutes followed by stretching |
| **Exercises:** | 38 minutes |

| | | | | Choose 1 exercise per row | | |
|---|---|---|---|---|---|---|
| **#** | **Muscle group** | **Reps** | **Sets\*** | **Barbell** | **Machine** | **Alternative** |
| 1 | Chest | 10-12 | 3 | Bench press | Chest press | Bench press (DB) |
| 2 | Back | 10-12 | 3 | Bent-over row | Seated row | One-arm row (DB) |
| 3 | Shoulders | 10-12 | 3 | Standing press | Shoulder press | Lateral raise (DB) |
| 4 | Front of arm | 10-12 | 3 | Biceps curl | Low-pulley curl | Biceps curl (DB) |
| 5 | Back of arm | 10-12 | 3 | Lying triceps extension | Triceps pushdown | Triceps kickback (DB) |
| 6 | Thighs | 10-12 | 3 | Lunge | Leg press | Squat (DB) |
| 7 | Core | 15-25 | 3 | Good morning | Abdominal crunch | Sit-up (BW) |

| | |
|---|---|
| **Rest period:** | 1 minute |
| **Cool-down:** | Slow walking for 5 minutes followed by stretching |
| **Workout tips:** | * At this point you should be able to perform the required three sets back to back. |

## WORKOUT 1

**Total time:** 51 minutes

**Weeks:** 1 and 2

**Days of the week:** Two nonconsecutive days*

**Warm-up:** Easy jogging or rope skipping for 5 minutes followed by stretching

**Upper-body exercises:** 21 minutes

|  |  |  |  | Choose 1 exercise per row | | |
| --- | --- | --- | --- | --- | --- | --- |
| # | Muscle group | Reps | Sets | Barbell | Machine | Alternative |
| 1 | Chest | 8-10 | 2** | Bench press | Chest press | Bench press (DB) |
| 2*** | Chest | 10-12 | 1 | Incline bench press | Pec deck | Chest fly (DB) |
| 3 | Back | 10-12 | 2 | Bent-over row | Seated row | One-arm row (DB) |
| 4 | Shoulders | 8-10 | 2** | Standing press | Shoulder press | Lateral raise (DB) |
| 5*** | Back | 10-12 | 1 | N/A | Lat pulldown | Double bent-over row (KB) |
| 6 | Back of arm | 10-12 | 2 | Lying triceps extension | Triceps pushdown | Triceps kickback (DB) |
| 7 | Front of arm | 10-12 | 2 | Biceps curl | Low-pulley curl | Biceps curl (DB) |

**Rest period:** 1 minute

**Cool-down:** Slow walking for 5 minutes followed by stretching

**Workout tips:** * When you make the change to four workouts per week, you will perform upper-body and lower-body workouts separately, allowing you to add new exercises and still complete your workouts in about the same time. A common program schedules upper-body exercises on Mondays and Thursdays and lower-body exercises on Tuesdays and Fridays.

** As you begin performing both sets with the heavier load (for fewer repetitions), you may have to decrease the load slightly in the second set to complete both sets in exercises 1 and 4.

*** Refer to chapter 4 to determine your starting loads for new exercises and chapter 6 to learn how to perform them correctly.

### WORKOUT 2

| | |
|---|---|
| **Total time:** | 44 minutes |
| **Weeks:** | 1 and 2 |
| **Days of the week:** | Two nonconsecutive days* |
| **Warm-up:** | Easy jogging or rope skipping for 5 minutes followed by stretching |
| **Lower-body exercises:** | 14 minutes |

| | | | | Choose 1 exercise per row | | |
|---|---|---|---|---|---|---|
| **#** | **Muscle group** | **Reps** | **Sets** | **Barbell** | **Machine** | **Alternative** |
| 1 | Thighs | 8-10 | 2** | Lunge | Leg press | Squat (DB) |
| 2*** | Thighs | 8-10 | 1 | Squat | Hip sled | Step-up (DB) |
| 3*** | Back of thigh | 10-12 | 1 | N/A | Leg (knee) curl | Leg curl (heel pull) (SB) |
| 4*** | Front of thigh | 10-12 | 1 | N/A | Leg (knee) extension | Wall squat (SB) |
| 5*** | Calf | 10-12 | 1 | Standing heel raise | Seated heel raise | One-leg standing heel raise (DB) |
| 6 | Core | 15-25 | 2 | Good morning | Abdominal crunch | Sit-up (BW) |

| | |
|---|---|
| **Rest period:** | 1 minute |
| **Cool-down:** | Slow walking for 5 minutes followed by stretching |
| **Workout tips:** | * When you make the change to four workouts per week, you will perform upper-body and lower-body workouts separately, allowing you to add new exercises and still complete your workouts in about the same time. A common program schedules upper-body exercises on Mondays and Thursdays and lower-body exercises on Tuesdays and Fridays. |
| | ** As you begin performing both sets with the heavier load (for fewer repetitions), you may have to decrease the load slightly in the second set to complete both sets in exercise 1. |
| | *** Refer to chapter 4 to determine your starting loads for new exercises and chapter 6 to learn how to perform them correctly. |

PURPLE ZONE

## WORKOUT 3

| | |
|---|---|
| **Total time:** | 55 minutes |
| **Weeks:** | 3 and 4 |
| **Days of the week:** | Two nonconsecutive days |
| **Warm-up:** | Easy jogging or rope skipping for 5 minutes followed by stretching |
| **Upper-body exercises:** | 25 minutes |

|  |  |  |  | Choose 1 exercise per row | | |
|---|---|---|---|---|---|---|
| **#** | **Muscle group** | **Reps** | **Sets** | **Barbell** | **Machine** | **Alternative** |
| 1 | Chest | 8-10 | 2 | Bench press | Chest press | Bench press (DB) |
| 2 | Chest | 10-12 | 2* | Incline bench press | Pec deck | Chest fly (DB) |
| 3 | Back | 10-12 | 2 | Bent-over row | Seated row | One-arm row (DB) |
| 4 | Shoulders | 8-10 | 2 | Standing press | Shoulder press | Lateral raise (DB) |
| 5 | Back | 10-12 | 2* | N/A | Lat pulldown | Double bent-over row (KB) |
| 6 | Back of arm | 10-12 | 2 | Lying triceps extension | Triceps pushdown | Triceps kickback (DB) |
| 7 | Front of arm | 10-12 | 2 | Biceps curl | Low-pulley curl | Biceps curl (DB) |

| | |
|---|---|
| **Rest period:** | 1 minute |
| **Cool-down:** | Slow walking for 5 minutes followed by stretching |
| **Workout tips:** | * You may need to readjust the loads that you are using in your new exercises to complete two back-to-back sets. |

## WORKOUT 4

| | |
|---|---|
| **Total time:** | 51 minutes |
| **Weeks:** | 3 and 4 |
| **Days of the week:** | Two nonconsecutive days |
| **Warm-up:** | Easy jogging or rope skipping for 5 minutes followed by stretching |
| **Lower-body exercises:** | 21 minutes |

| | | | | Choose 1 exercise per row | | |
|---|---|---|---|---|---|---|
| **#** | **Muscle group** | **Reps** | **Sets** | **Barbell** | **Machine** | **Alternative** |
| 1 | Thighs | 8-10 | 2 | Lunge | Leg press | Squat (DB) |
| 2 | Thighs | 8-10 | 2* | Squat | Hip sled | Step-up (DB) |
| 3 | Back of thigh | 10-12 | 2* | N/A | Leg (knee) curl | Leg curl (heel pull) (SB) |
| 4 | Front of thigh | 10-12 | 2* | N/A | Leg (knee) extension | Wall squat (SB) |
| 5 | Calf | 10-12 | 2* | Standing heel raise | Seated heel raise | One-leg standing heel raise (DB) |
| 6 | Core | 15-25 | 2 | Good morning | Abdominal crunch | Sit-up (BW) |

| | |
|---|---|
| **Rest period:** | 1 minute |
| **Cool-down:** | Slow walking for 5 minutes followed by stretching |
| **Workout tips:** | * You may need to readjust the loads that you are using in your new exercises to complete two back-to-back sets. |

## WORKOUT 5

| | | |
|---|---|---|
| **Total time:** | | 58 minutes |
| **Weeks:** | | 5 and 6 |
| **Days of the week:** | | Two nonconsecutive days |
| **Warm-up:** | | Easy jogging or rope skipping for 5 minutes followed by stretching |

**Upper-body exercises:** 28 minutes

| | | | | Choose 1 exercise per row | | |
|---|---|---|---|---|---|---|
| **#** | **Muscle group** | **Reps** | **Sets** | **Barbell** | **Machine** | **Alternative** |
| 1 | Chest | 8-10 | 3* | Bench press | Chest press | Bench press (DB) |
| 2 | Chest | 10-12 | 2 | Incline bench press | Pec deck | Chest fly (DB) |
| 3 | Back | 10-12 | 2 | Bent-over row | Seated row | One-arm row (DB) |
| 4 | Shoulders | 8-10 | 3* | Standing press | Shoulder press | Lateral raise (DB) |
| 5 | Back | 10-12 | 2 | N/A | Lat pulldown | Double bent-over row (KB) |
| 6 | Back of arm | 10-12 | 2 | Lying triceps extension | Triceps pushdown | Triceps kickback (DB) |
| 7 | Front of arm | 10-12 | 2 | Biceps curl | Low-pulley curl | Biceps curl (DB) |

| | | |
|---|---|---|
| **Rest period:** | | 1 minute |
| **Cool-down:** | | Slow walking for 5 minutes followed by stretching |
| **Workout tips:** | | * To increase the difficulty of exercises 1 and 4, keep readjusting the load to perform 8 repetitions per set instead of 10. To do this, apply the two-for-two rule (see chapter 13) when you reach 10 repetitions in the last set for two consecutive workouts. |

PURPLE ZONE

## WORKOUT 6

| | |
|---|---|
| **Total time:** | 54 minutes |
| **Weeks:** | 5 and 6 |
| **Days of the week:** | Two nonconsecutive days |
| **Warm-up:** | Easy jogging or rope skipping for 5 minutes followed by stretching |
| **Lower-body exercises:** | 24 minutes |

| | | | | Choose 1 exercise per row | | |
|---|---|---|---|---|---|---|
| **#** | **Muscle group** | **Reps** | **Sets** | **Barbell** | **Machine** | **Alternative** |
| 1 | Thighs | 8-10 | 3* | Lunge | Leg press | Squat (DB) |
| 2 | Thighs | 8-10 | 3* | Squat | Hip sled | Step-up (DB) |
| 3 | Back of thigh | 10-12 | 2 | N/A | Leg (knee) curl | Leg curl (heel pull) (SB) |
| 4 | Front of thigh | 10-12 | 2 | N/A | Leg (knee) extension | Wall squat (SB) |
| 5 | Calf | 10-12 | 2 | Standing heel raise | Seated heel raise | One-leg standing heel raise (DB) |
| 6 | Core | 15-25 | 3 | Good morning | Abdominal crunch | Sit-up (BW) |

| | |
|---|---|
| **Rest period:** | 1 minute |
| **Cool-down:** | Slow walking for 5 minutes followed by stretching |
| **Workout tips:** | * To increase the difficulty of exercises 1 and 2, keep readjusting the load to perform 8 repetitions per set instead of 10. To do this, apply the two-for-two rule (see chapter 13) when you reach 10 repetitions in the last set for two consecutive workouts. |

# 10

# Yellow Zone

The Yellow Zone is for you if you have been weight training recently on a consistent basis and scored in the average fitness classification from chapter 3, or if you completed the Purple Zone and are looking for a more advanced program. The workouts in this zone will help you prepare for more intense workouts in the upcoming zones.

## Zone Highlights

The Yellow Zone covers multiple two-week workouts for each training outcome. With the exception of the first two weeks of the muscle toning workouts, all of the other workouts in this zone have additional upper-body and lower-body exercises beyond the foundational exercises for each of the seven major muscle groups.

If you do not have the necessary equipment or you do not feel comfortable or experienced enough to perform any of the three exercises listed for a muscle group, go to the exercise finder in chapter 6 to choose a replacement exercise for the same muscle group. Further, if you want some variety at any point in your program, you can also find a replacement exercise as long as it trains the same muscle group. Be aware, though, that your strength will not be the same because you are not used to performing the new exercise. Use the guidelines in chapter 4 to determine your starting load and then adjust that load using tables 4.10 or 4.11 to match the number of repetitions (e.g., 6-8, 8-10, or 10-12 rather than 12-15) that is listed in your zone workout table for that muscle group.

### Muscle Toning

- The first two weeks require three sets of 12 to 15 repetitions in all seven exercises for three workouts a week.
- Weeks 3 through 6 include three additional exercises—one set of 12 to 15 repetitions each for your chest, back, and calves. To determine what loads you should use in the new exercises, follow the guidelines in chapter 4.

## Body Shaping

- A major change in this zone is that you will be completing four work-outs each week; your program is divided into two upper-body and two lower-body training days. Because of the increase in the number of weekly workouts, weeks 1 and 2 will require only one set of 10 to 12 repetitions in the two new upper-body exercises and the four new lower-body exercises. The upper-body exercises include two each for the chest and back and one each for the shoulders, front of upper arm (biceps), and back of upper arm (triceps). The lower-body exercises include two for the thighs and one each for the back of thigh (ham-strings), front of thigh (quadriceps), calves, and core. Chapter 4 will help you determine the loads for your new exercises.
- Weeks 3 through 6 gradually return you to three back-to-back sets in each of your seven upper-body and six lower-body exercises.

## Strength Training

- Weeks 1 and 2 add more sets (now you will be doing three) in the exercises that you were performing only two sets of at the end of the Purple Zone.
- Weeks 3 and 4 add more sets (now you will be doing four) in the two major upper-body exercises and the first lower-body thigh exercise. These three exercises are MJEs that you will use to build strength during the rest of this zone and on through the Red Zone.
- At week 5, the strength training program makes another increase in training intensity. Depending on the exercise, the program now has different repetition goals: 6 to 8 repetitions for the MJEs and 8 to 10 or 10 to 12 repetitions for all others. In addition, you will begin per-forming weight training exercises as part of your warm-up. Follow the warm-up procedure outlined in the warm-up section of each strength training workout (those sets are not counted in the number of sets that the program requires you to complete).
- Remember to increase the weight for the MJEs when you begin per-forming 6 to 8 repetitions per set.

## WORKOUT 1

| | |
|---|---|
| **Total time:** | 1 hour, 2 minutes |
| **Weeks:** | 1 and 2 |
| **Days of the week:** | Three nonconsecutive days |
| **Warm-up:** | Easy jogging or rope skipping for 5 minutes followed by stretching |
| **Exercises:** | 32 minutes |

| | | | | Choose 1 exercise per row | | |
|---|---|---|---|---|---|---|
| **#** | **Muscle group** | **Reps** | **Sets** | **Barbell** | **Machine** | **Alternative** |
| 1 | Chest | 12-15 | 3 | Bench press | Chest press | Bench press (DB) |
| 2 | Back | 12-15 | 3 | Bent-over row | Seated row | One-arm row (DB) |
| 3 | Shoulders | 12-15 | 3 | Standing press | Shoulder press | Lateral raise (DB) |
| 4 | Front of arm | 12-15 | 3 | Biceps curl | Low-pulley curl | Biceps curl (DB) |
| 5 | Back of arm | 12-15 | 3 | Lying triceps extension | Triceps pushdown | Triceps kickback (DB) |
| 6 | Thighs | 12-15 | 3 | Lunge | Leg press | Squat (DB) |
| 7 | Core | 15-25 | 3 | Good morning | Abdominal crunch | Sit-up (BW) |

| | |
|---|---|
| **Rest period:** | 30 seconds* |
| **Cool-down:** | Slow walking for 5 minutes followed by stretching |
| **Workout tips:** | * You can add a challenging element to your program as your training status improves by slightly decreasing the rest time to 20 seconds between sets or exercises. |

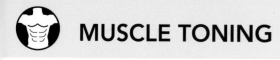
## WORKOUT 2

| | |
|---|---|
| **Total time:** | 1 hour, 6 minutes |
| **Weeks:** | 3 and 4 |
| **Days of the week:** | Three nonconsecutive days |
| **Warm-up:** | Easy jogging or rope skipping for 5 minutes followed by stretching |
| **Exercises:** | 36 minutes |

| | | | | Choose 1 exercise per row | | |
|---|---|---|---|---|---|---|
| # | Muscle group | Reps | Sets | Barbell | Machine | Alternative |
| 1 | Chest | 12-15 | 3 | Bench press | Chest press | Bench press (DB) |
| 2* | Chest | 12-15 | 1** | Incline bench press | Pec deck | Chest fly (DB) |
| 3 | Back | 12-15 | 3 | Bent-over row | Seated row | One-arm row (DB) |
| 4 | Shoulders | 12-15 | 3 | Standing press | Shoulder press | Lateral raise (DB) |
| 5* | Back | 12-15 | 1** | N/A | Lat pulldown | Double bent-over row (KB) |
| 6 | Back of arm | 12-15 | 3 | Lying triceps extension | Triceps pushdown | Overhead triceps extension (DB) |
| 7 | Front of arm | 12-15 | 3 | Biceps curl | Low-pulley curl | Biceps curl (DB) |
| 8 | Thighs | 12-15 | 3 | Lunge | Leg press | Squat (DB) |
| 9 | Core | 15-25 | 3 | Good morning | Abdominal crunch | Sit-up (BW) |
| 10* | Calf | 12-15 | 1** | Standing heel raise | Seated heel raise | One-leg standing heel raise (DB) |

| | |
|---|---|
| **Rest period:** | 30 seconds |
| **Cool-down:** | Slow walking for 5 minutes followed by stretching |
| **Workout tips:** | * Now you are completing 10 exercises per session; to learn how to perform your new exercises, consult chapter 6. The procedure described in chapter 4 will help you determine your starting loads in these exercises. |
| | ** For these two weeks, perform the one set of exercises 2, 5, and 10 after completing all the other exercises. |

## WORKOUT 3

**Total time:**          1 hour, 6 minutes

**Weeks:**               5 and 6

**Days of the week:**    Three nonconsecutive days

**Warm-up:**             Easy jogging or rope skipping for 5 minutes followed by stretching

**Exercises:**           36 minutes

| | | | | Choose 1 exercise per row | | |
|---|---|---|---|---|---|---|
| #* | Muscle group | Reps | Sets | Barbell | Machine | Alternative |
| 1 | Chest | 12-15 | 3 | Bench press | Chest press | Bench press (DB) |
| 2 | Chest | 12-15 | 1 | Incline bench press | Pec deck | Chest fly (DB) |
| 3 | Back | 12-15 | 3 | Bent-over row | Seated row | One-arm row (DB) |
| 4 | Shoulders | 12-15 | 3 | Standing press | Shoulder press | Lateral raise (DB) |
| 5 | Back | 12-15 | 1 | N/A | Lat pulldown | Double bent-over row (KB) |
| 6 | Back of arm | 12-15 | 3 | Lying triceps extension | Triceps pushdown | Overhead triceps extension (DB) |
| 7 | Front of arm | 12-15 | 3 | Biceps curl | Low-pulley curl | Biceps curl (DB) |
| 8 | Thighs | 12-15 | 3 | Lunge | Leg press | Squat (DB) |
| 9 | Core | 15-25 | 3 | Good morning | Abdominal crunch | Sit-up (BW) |
| 10 | Calf | 12-15 | 1 | Standing heel raise | Seated heel raise | One-leg standing heel raise (DB) |

**Rest period:**     30 seconds

**Cool-down:**      Slow walking for 5 minutes followed by stretching

**Workout tips:**   * Perform all exercises in the order listed.

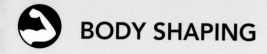

# BODY SHAPING

## WORKOUT 1

| | |
|---|---|
| **Total time:** | 1 hour, 1 minute |
| **Weeks:** | 1 and 2 |
| **Days of the week:** | Two nonconsecutive days* |
| **Warm-up:** | Easy jogging or rope skipping for 5 minutes followed by stretching |
| **Upper-body exercises:** | 31 minutes |

| # | Muscle group | Reps | Sets | Barbell | Machine | Alternative |
|---|---|---|---|---|---|---|
| | | | | | | **Choose 1 exercise per row** |
| 1 | Chest | 10-12 | 3 | Bench press | Chest press | Bench press (DB) |
| 2** | Chest | 10-12 | 1 | Incline bench press | Pec deck | Chest fly (DB) |
| 3 | Back | 10-12 | 3 | Bent-over row | Seated row | One-arm row (DB) |
| 4 | Shoulders | 10-12 | 3 | Standing press | Shoulder press | Lateral raise (DB) |
| 5** | Back | 10-12 | 1 | N/A | Lat pulldown | Double bent-over row (KB) |
| 6 | Back of arm | 10-12 | 3 | Lying triceps extension | Triceps pushdown | Triceps kickback (DB) |
| 7 | Front of arm | 10-12 | 3 | Biceps curl | Low-pulley curl | Biceps curl (DB) |

| | |
|---|---|
| **Rest period:** | 1 minute |
| **Cool-down:** | Slow walking for 5 minutes followed by stretching |
| **Workout tips:** | * When you make the change to four workouts per week, you will perform upper-body and lower-body workouts separately, allowing you to add new exercises and still complete your workouts in about the same time. A common program schedules upper-body exercises on Mondays and Thursdays and lower-body exercises on Tuesdays and Fridays. |
| | ** Refer to chapter 4 to determine your starting loads for new exercises and chapter 6 to learn how to perform them correctly. |

## WORKOUT 2

| | |
|---|---|
| **Total time:** | 48 minutes |
| **Weeks:** | 1 and 2 |
| **Days of the week:** | Two nonconsecutive days* |
| **Warm-up:** | Easy jogging or rope skipping for 5 minutes followed by stretching |
| **Lower-body exercises:** | 18 minutes |

| | | | | Choose 1 exercise per row | | |
|---|---|---|---|---|---|---|
| **#** | **Muscle group** | **Reps** | **Sets** | **Barbell** | **Machine** | **Alternative** |
| 1** | Thighs | 10-12 | 1 | Lunge | Leg press | Squat (DB) |
| 2 | Thighs | 10-12 | 3 | Squat | Hip sled | Step-up (DB) |
| 3** | Back of thigh | 10-12 | 1 | N/A | Leg (knee) curl | Leg curl (heel pull) (SB) |
| 4** | Front of thigh | 10-12 | 1 | N/A | Leg (knee) extension | Wall squat (SB) |
| 5** | Calf | 10-12 | 1 | Standing heel raise | Seated heel raise | One-leg standing heel raise (DB) |
| 6 | Core | 15-25 | 3 | Good morning | Abdominal crunch | Sit-up (BW) |

| | |
|---|---|
| **Rest period:** | 1 minute |
| **Cool-down:** | Slow walking for 5 minutes followed by stretching |
| **Workout tips:** | * When you make the change to four workouts per week, you will perform upper-body and lower-body workouts separately, allowing you to add new exercises and still complete your workouts in about the same time. A common program schedules upper-body exercises on Mondays and Thursdays and lower-body exercises on Tuesdays and Fridays. |
| | ** Refer to chapter 4 to determine your starting loads for new exercises and chapter 6 to learn how to perform them correctly. |

YELLOW ZONE

## WORKOUT 3

| | |
|---|---|
| **Total time:** | 1 hour, 4 minutes |
| **Weeks:** | 3 and 4 |
| **Days of the week:** | Two nonconsecutive days |
| **Warm-up:** | Easy jogging or rope skipping for 5 minutes followed by stretching |
| **Upper-body exercises:** | 34 minutes |

| | | | | Choose 1 exercise per row | | |
|---|---|---|---|---|---|---|
| # | Muscle group | Reps | Sets | Barbell | Machine | Alternative |
| 1 | Chest | 10-12 | 3 | Bench press | Chest press | Bench press (DB) |
| 2 | Chest | 10-12 | 2* | Incline bench press | Pec deck | Chest fly (DB) |
| 3 | Back | 10-12 | 3 | Bent-over row | Seated row | One-arm row (DB) |
| 4 | Shoulders | 10-12 | 3 | Standing press | Shoulder press | Lateral raise (DB) |
| 5 | Back | 10-12 | 2* | N/A | Lat pulldown | Double bent-over row (KB) |
| 6 | Back of arm | 10-12 | 3 | Lying triceps extension | Triceps pushdown | Triceps kickback (DB) |
| 7 | Front of arm | 10-12 | 3 | Biceps curl | Low-pulley curl | Biceps curl (DB) |

| | |
|---|---|
| **Rest period:** | 1 minute |
| **Cool-down:** | Slow walking for 5 minutes followed by stretching |
| **Workout tips:** | * Be sure to perform the sets for exercises 2 and 5 back to back and in the order listed. |

## WORKOUT 4

| | |
|---|---|
| **Total time:** | 55 minutes |
| **Weeks:** | 3 and 4 |
| **Days of the week:** | Two nonconsecutive days |
| **Warm-up:** | Easy jogging or rope skipping for 5 minutes followed by stretching |
| **Lower-body exercises:** | 25 minutes |

| | | | | Choose 1 exercise per row | | |
|---|---|---|---|---|---|---|
| **#** | **Muscle group** | **Reps** | **Sets** | **Barbell** | **Machine** | **Alternative** |
| 1 | Thighs | 10-12 | 2* | Lunge | Leg press | Squat (DB) |
| 2 | Thighs | 10-12 | 3 | Squat | Hip sled | Step-up (DB) |
| 3 | Back of thigh | 10-12 | 2* | N/A | Leg (knee) curl | Leg curl (heel pull) (SB) |
| 4 | Front of thigh | 10-12 | 2* | N/A | Leg (knee) extension | Wall squat (SB) |
| 5 | Calf | 10-12 | 2* | Standing heel raise | Seated heel raise | One-leg standing heel raise (DB) |
| 6 | Core | 15-25 | 3 | Good morning | Abdominal crunch | Sit-up (BW) |

| | |
|---|---|
| **Rest period:** | 1 minute |
| **Cool-down:** | Slow walking for 5 minutes followed by stretching |
| **Workout tips:** | * Be sure to perform the sets for exercises 1, 3, 4, and 5 back to back and in the order listed. |

## WORKOUT 5

| | |
|---|---|
| **Total time:** | 1 hour, 8 minutes |
| **Weeks:** | 5 and 6 |
| **Days of the week:** | Two nonconsecutive days |
| **Warm-up:** | Easy jogging or rope skipping for 5 minutes followed by stretching |
| **Upper-body exercises:** | 38 minutes |

| | | | | Choose 1 exercise per row | | |
|---|---|---|---|---|---|---|
| # | Muscle group | Reps | Sets | Barbell | Machine | Alternative |
| 1 | Chest | 10-12 | 3 | Bench press | Chest press | Bench press (DB) |
| 2 | Chest | 10-12 | 3* | Incline bench press | Pec deck | Chest fly (DB) |
| 3 | Back | 10-12 | 3 | Bent-over row | Seated row | One-arm row (DB) |
| 4 | Shoulders | 10-12 | 3 | Standing press | Shoulder press | Lateral raise (DB) |
| 5 | Back | 10-12 | 3* | N/A | Lat pulldown | Double bent-over row (KB) |
| 6 | Back of arm | 10-12 | 3 | Lying triceps extension | Triceps pushdown | Triceps kickback (DB) |
| 7 | Front of arm | 10-12 | 3 | Biceps curl | Low-pulley curl | Biceps curl (DB) |

| | |
|---|---|
| **Rest period:** | 1 minute |
| **Cool-down:** | Slow walking for 5 minutes followed by stretching |
| **Workout tips:** | * Be sure to perform the sets for exercises 2 and 5 back to back and in the order listed. |

## WORKOUT 6

| | |
|---|---|
| **Total time:** | 1 hour, 2 minutes |
| **Weeks:** | 5 and 6 |
| **Days of the week:** | Two nonconsecutive days |
| **Warm-up:** | Easy jogging or rope skipping for 5 minutes followed by stretching |
| **Lower-body exercises:** | 32 minutes |

| | | | | Choose 1 exercise per row | | |
|---|---|---|---|---|---|---|
| **#** | **Muscle group** | **Reps** | **Sets** | **Barbell** | **Machine** | **Alternative** |
| 1 | Thighs | 10-12 | 3* | Lunge | Leg press | Squat (DB) |
| 2 | Thighs | 10-12 | 3 | Squat | Hip sled | Step-up (DB) |
| 3 | Back of thigh | 10-12 | 3* | N/A | Leg (knee) curl | Leg curl (heel pull) (SB) |
| 4 | Front of thigh | 10-12 | 3* | N/A | Leg (knee) extension | Wall squat (SB) |
| 5 | Calf | 10-12 | 3* | Standing heel raise | Seated heel raise | One-leg standing heel raise (DB) |
| 6 | Core | 15-25 | 3 | Good morning | Abdominal crunch | Sit-up (BW) |

| | |
|---|---|
| **Rest period:** | 1 minute |
| **Cool-down:** | Slow walking for 5 minutes followed by stretching |
| **Workout tips:** | * Be sure to perform the sets for exercises 1, 3, 4, and 5 back to back and in the order listed. |

# STRENGTH TRAINING

## WORKOUT 1

| | | |
|---|---|---|
| **Total time:** | 1 hour, 17 minutes |
| **Weeks:** | 1 and 2 |
| **Days of the week:** | Two nonconsecutive days |
| **Warm-up:** | Easy jogging or rope skipping for 5 minutes followed by stretching |
| **Upper-body exercises:** | 37 minutes |

| | | | | Choose 1 exercise per row | | |
|---|---|---|---|---|---|---|
| # | Muscle group | Reps | Sets* | Barbell | Machine | Alternative |
| 1** | Chest | 8-10 | 3 | Bench press | Chest press | Bench press (DB) |
| 2 | Chest | 10-12 | 3 | Incline bench press | Pec deck | Chest fly (DB) |
| 3 | Back | 10-12 | 3 | Bent-over row | Seated row | One-arm row (DB) |
| 4** | Shoulders | 8-10 | 3 | Standing press | Shoulder press | Lateral raise (DB) |
| 5 | Back | 10-12 | 3 | N/A | Lat pulldown | Double bent-over row (KB) |
| 6 | Back of arm | 10-12 | 3 | Lying triceps extension | Triceps pushdown | Triceps kickback (DB) |
| 7 | Front of arm | 10-12 | 3 | Biceps curl | Low-pulley curl | Biceps curl (DB) |

| | |
|---|---|
| **Rest period:** | 1 minute |
| **Cool-down:** | Slow walking for 5 minutes followed by stretching |
| **Workout tips:** | * You may need to readjust the loads to complete three back-to-back sets. |
| | ** As the loads become heavier, remember to use a spotter, especially for the barbell and dumbbell versions of exercises 1 and 4. |

## WORKOUT 2

| | |
|---|---|
| **Total time:** | 1 hour, 2 minutes |
| **Weeks:** | 1 and 2 |
| **Days of the week:** | Two nonconsecutive days |
| **Warm-up:** | Easy jogging or rope skipping for 5 minutes followed by stretching |
| **Lower-body exercises:** | 32 minutes |

| | | | | Choose 1 exercise per row | | |
|---|---|---|---|---|---|---|
| # | Muscle group | Reps | Sets* | Barbell | Machine | Alternative |
| 1** | Thighs | 8-10 | 3 | Lunge | Leg press | Squat (DB) |
| 2** | Thighs | 8-10 | 3 | Squat | Hip sled | Step-up (DB) |
| 3 | Back of thigh | 10-12 | 3 | N/A | Leg (knee) curl | Leg curl (heel pull) (SB) |
| 4 | Front of thigh | 10-12 | 3 | N/A | Leg (knee) extension | Wall squat (SB) |
| 5 | Calf | 10-12 | 3 | Standing heel raise | Seated heel raise | One-leg standing heel raise (DB) |
| 6 | Core | 15-25 | 3 | Good morning | Abdominal crunch | Sit-up (BW) |

| | |
|---|---|
| **Rest period:** | 1 minute |
| **Cool-down:** | Slow walking for 5 minutes followed by stretching |
| **Workout tips:** | * You may need to readjust the loads to complete three back-to-back sets. |
| | ** As the loads become heavier, remember to use a spotter, especially for the barbell and dumbbell versions of exercises 1 and 2. |

YELLOW ZONE

### WORKOUT 3

| | |
|---|---|
| **Total time:** | 1 hour, 10 minutes |
| **Weeks:** | 3 and 4 |
| **Days of the week:** | Two nonconsecutive days |
| **Warm-up:** | Easy jogging or rope skipping for 5 minutes followed by stretching |
| **Upper-body exercises:** | 40 minutes |

| | | | | Choose 1 exercise per row | | |
|---|---|---|---|---|---|---|
| **#** | **Muscle group** | **Reps** | **Sets** | **Barbell** | **Machine** | **Alternative** |
| 1 | Chest | 8-10 | 4* | Bench press | Chest press | Bench press (DB) |
| 2 | Chest | 10-12 | 3 | Incline bench press | Pec deck | Chest fly (DB) |
| 3 | Back | 10-12 | 3 | Bent-over row | Seated row | One-arm row (DB) |
| 4 | Shoulders | 8-10 | 4* | Standing press | Shoulder press | Lateral raise (DB) |
| 5 | Back | 10-12 | 3 | N/A | Lat pulldown | Double bent-over row (KB) |
| 6 | Back of arm | 10-12 | 3 | Lying triceps extension | Triceps pushdown | Triceps kickback (DB) |
| 7 | Front of arm | 10-12 | 3 | Biceps curl | Low-pulley curl | Biceps curl (DB) |

| | |
|---|---|
| **Rest period:** | 1 minute |
| **Cool-down:** | Slow walking for 5 minutes followed by stretching |
| **Workout tips:** | * As you begin performing four sets in exercises 1 and 4, you may have to decrease the load by 5 pounds (~2.5 kg) to complete all four sets. |

## WORKOUT 4

| | |
|---|---|
| **Total time:** | 1 hour, 3 minutes |
| **Weeks:** | 3 and 4 |
| **Days of the week**: | Two nonconsecutive days |
| **Warm-up:** | Easy jogging or rope skipping for 5 minutes followed by stretching |
| **Lower-body exercises:** | 33 minutes |

| # | Muscle group | Reps | Sets | Choose 1 exercise per row | | |
|---|---|---|---|---|---|---|
| | | | | **Barbell** | **Machine** | **Alternative** |
| 1 | Thighs | 8-10 | 4* | Lunge | Leg press | Squat (DB) |
| 2 | Thighs | 8-10 | 3 | Squat | Hip sled | Step-up (DB) |
| 3 | Back of thigh | 10-12 | 3 | N/A | Leg (knee) curl | Leg curl (heel pull) (SB) |
| 4 | Front of thigh | 10-12 | 3 | N/A | Leg (knee) extension | Wall squat (SB) |
| 5 | Calf | 10-12 | 3 | Standing heel raise | Seated heel raise | One-leg standing heel raise (DB) |
| 6 | Core | 15-25 | 3 | Good morning | Abdominal crunch | Sit-up (BW) |

| | |
|---|---|
| **Rest period:** | 1 minute |
| **Cool-down:** | Slow walking for 5 minutes followed by stretching |
| **Workout tips:** | * As you begin performing four sets in exercise 1, you may have to decrease the load by 10 pounds (~5 kg) to complete all four sets. |

## WORKOUT 5

| | |
|---|---|
| **Total time:** | 1 hour, 16 minutes |
| **Weeks:** | 5 and 6 |
| **Days of the week:** | Two nonconsecutive days |
| **Warm-up:** | Easy jogging or rope skipping for 5 minutes followed by stretching. Before performing your first set of exercises 1 and 4, do one warm-up set of 8 to 10 repetitions with half to three-quarters of the load that you typically use for that exercise. Rest 1 to 2 minutes before starting your scheduled sets. |

**Upper-body exercises:** 46 minutes

| | | | | Choose 1 exercise per row | | |
|---|---|---|---|---|---|---|
| **#** | **Muscle group** | **Reps** | **Sets** | **Barbell** | **Machine** | **Alternative** |
| 1** | Chest | 6-8* | 3 | Bench press | Chest press | Bench press (DB) |
| 2 | Chest | 10-12 | 3 | Incline bench press | Pec deck | Chest fly (DB) |
| 3 | Back | 10-12 | 3 | Bent-over row | Seated row | One-arm row (DB) |
| 4** | Shoulders | 6-8* | 3 | Standing press | Shoulder press | Lateral raise (DB) |
| 5 | Back | 10-12 | 3 | N/A | Lat pulldown | Double bent-over row (KB) |
| 6 | Back of arm | 10-12 | 3 | Lying triceps extension | Triceps pushdown | Triceps kickback (DB) |
| 7 | Front of arm | 10-12 | 3 | Biceps curl | Low-pulley curl | Biceps curl (DB) |

| | |
|---|---|
| **Rest period:** | 2 minutes for exercises 1 and 4**; 1 minute for all others |
| **Cool-down:** | Slow walking for 5 minutes followed by stretching |
| **Workout tips:** | * In exercises 1 and 4 you will perform 6 to 8 repetitions. To do this, add 5 to 10 pounds (~2.5-5 kg) to the loads from workout 3 of this zone or consult chapter 4 for a more specific method of determining new loads. |
| | ** Notice that the heavier sets of 6 to 8 repetitions require more rest between sets and a spotter for the barbell and dumbbell versions of exercises 1 and 4. |

## WORKOUT 6

| | |
|---|---|
| **Total time:** | 1 hour, 6 minutes |
| **Weeks:** | 5 and 6 |
| **Days of the week:** | Two nonconsecutive days |
| **Warm-up:** | Easy jogging or rope skipping for 5 minutes followed by stretching. Before performing your first set of exercise 1, do one warm-up set of 8 to 10 repetitions with half to three-quarters of the load that you typically use for that exercise. Rest 1 to 2 minutes before starting your scheduled sets. |

**Lower-body exercises:** 36 minutes

| | | | | Choose 1 exercise per row | | |
|---|---|---|---|---|---|---|
| # | Muscle group | Reps | Sets | Barbell | Machine | Alternative |
| 1** | Thighs | 6-8* | 3 | Lunge | Leg press | Squat (DB) |
| 2** | Thighs | 8-10 | 3 | Squat | Hip sled | Step-up (DB) |
| 3 | Back of thigh | 10-12 | 3 | N/A | Leg (knee) curl | Leg curl (heel pull) (SB) |
| 4 | Front of thigh | 10-12 | 3 | N/A | Leg (knee) extension | Wall squat (SB) |
| 5 | Calf | 10-12 | 3 | Standing heel raise | Seated heel raise | One-leg standing heel raise (DB) |
| 6 | Core | 15-25 | 3 | Good morning | Abdominal crunch | Sit-up (BW) |

| | |
|---|---|
| **Rest period:** | 2 minutes for exercise 1**; 1 minute for all others |
| **Cool-down:** | Slow walking for 5 minutes followed by stretching |
| **Workout tips:** | * In exercise 1 you will perform 6 to 8 repetitions. To do this, add 10 to 20 pounds (~5-10 kg) to the loads from workout 4 of this zone or consult chapter 4 for a more specific method of determining new loads. |
| | ** Notice that the heavier sets of 6 to 8 repetitions require more rest between sets and a spotter for the barbell and dumbbell versions of exercises 1 and 2. |

YELLOW ZONE

# Orange Zone

# 11

The Orange Zone is for you if you have not been weight training recently on a consistent basis and scored in the high fitness classification from chapter 3, or if you completed the Yellow Zone and are looking for a more advanced program. The workouts in this zone are very intense and require dedication if you want to be successful.

## Zone Highlights

The Orange Zone covers multiple two-week workouts for each training outcome. All of the workouts in this zone have additional upper-body and lower-body exercises beyond the foundational exercises for each of the seven major muscle groups.

If you do not have the necessary equipment or you do not feel comfortable or experienced enough to perform any of the three exercises listed for a muscle group, go to the exercise finder in chapter 6 to choose a replacement exercise for the same muscle group. Further, if you want some variety at any point in your program, you can also find a replacement exercise as long as it trains the same muscle group. Be aware, though, that your strength will not be the same because you are not used to performing the new exercise. Use the guidelines in chapter 4 to determine your starting load and then adjust that load using tables 4.10 or 4.11 to match the number of repetitions (e.g., 4-6, 6-8, 8-10, or 10-12 rather than 12-15) that is listed in your zone workout table for that muscle group.

### Muscle Toning

Weeks 1 and 2 require only two sets in the three additional exercises; by the start of week 3 you will be completing three sets in all 10 exercises. The final two weeks add one set (now you will be doing four) in the seven original exercises.

## Body Shaping

- For your upper-body workouts, weeks 1 and 2 add three exercises— one set of 10 to 12 repetitions each for your shoulders, front of upper arm (biceps), and back of upper arm (triceps).
- For your lower-body workouts, weeks 1 and 2 add two exercises—one set of 10 to 12 repetitions each for your thighs and calves.
- To determine what loads you should use in the new exercises, follow the guidelines in chapter 4.
- Weeks 3 through 6 gradually add sets so that you finish this zone with three back-to-back sets in each of your 10 upper-body and 8 lower-body exercises.

## Strength Training

- Weeks 1 and 2 add one set (now you will be doing four) to the three MJEs (two for the upper body and one for the lower body).
- For weeks 3 and 4, the MJEs now require you to perform only 4 to 6 repetitions, but you use a heavier weight. Because of this increase, you need to complete only three sets per MJE.
- Weeks 5 and 6 gradually return you to four sets in each MJE.

## WORKOUT 1

**Total time:**     1 hour, 11 minutes

**Weeks:**     1 and 2

**Days of the week:**     Three nonconsecutive days

**Warm-up:**     Easy jogging or rope skipping for 5 minutes followed by stretching

**Exercises:**     41 minutes

| | | | | Choose 1 exercise per row | | |
|---|---|---|---|---|---|---|
| # | Muscle group | Reps | Sets | Barbell | Machine | Alternative |
| 1 | Chest | 12-15 | 3 | Bench press | Chest press | Bench press (DB) |
| 2 | Chest | 12-15 | 2* | Incline bench press | Pec deck | Chest fly (DB) |
| 3 | Back | 12-15 | 3 | Bent-over row | Seated row | One-arm row (DB) |
| 4 | Shoulders | 12-15 | 3 | Standing press | Shoulder press | Lateral raise (DB) |
| 5 | Back | 12-15 | 2* | N/A | Lat pulldown | Double bent-over row (KB) |
| 6 | Back of arm | 12-15 | 3 | Lying triceps extension | Triceps pushdown | Overhead triceps extension (DB) |
| 7 | Front of arm | 12-15 | 3 | Biceps curl | Low-pulley curl | Biceps curl (DB) |
| 8 | Thighs | 12-15 | 3 | Lunge | Leg press | Squat (DB) |
| 9 | Core | 15-25 | 3 | Good morning | Abdominal crunch | Sit-up (BW) |
| 10 | Calf | 12-15 | 2* | Standing heel raise | Seated heel raise | One-leg standing heel raise (DB) |

**Rest period:**     30 seconds

**Cool-down:**     Slow walking for 5 minutes followed by stretching

**Workout tips:**     * At this point, you should be able to perform the required two sets back to back.

ORANGE ZONE

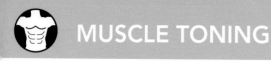
## WORKOUT 2

| | | |
|---|---|---|
| **Total time:** | | 1 hour, 15 minutes |
| **Weeks:** | | 3 and 4 |
| **Days of the week:** | | Three nonconsecutive days |
| **Warm-up:** | | Easy jogging or rope skipping for 5 minutes followed by stretching |
| **Exercises:** | | 45 minutes |

| | | | | Choose 1 exercise per row | | |
|---|---|---|---|---|---|---|
| **#** | **Muscle group** | **Reps** | **Sets** | **Barbell** | **Machine** | **Alternative** |
| 1 | Chest | 12-15 | 3 | Bench press | Chest press | Bench press (DB) |
| 2 | Chest | 12-15 | 3* | Incline bench press | Pec deck | Chest fly (DB) |
| 3 | Back | 12-15 | 3 | Bent-over row | Seated row | One-arm row (DB) |
| 4 | Shoulders | 12-15 | 3 | Standing press | Shoulder press | Lateral raise (DB) |
| 5 | Back | 12-15 | 3 | N/A | Lat pulldown | Double bent-over row (KB) |
| 6 | Back of arm | 12-15 | 3 | Lying triceps extension | Triceps pushdown | Overhead triceps extension (DB) |
| 7 | Front of arm | 12-15 | 3 | Biceps curl | Low-pulley curl | Biceps curl (DB) |
| 8 | Thighs | 12-15 | 3 | Lunge | Leg press | Squat (DB) |
| 9 | Core | 15-25 | 3 | Good morning | Abdominal crunch | Sit-up (BW) |
| 10 | Calf | 12-15 | 3 | Standing heel raise | Seated heel raise | One-leg standing heel raise (DB) |

| | |
|---|---|
| **Rest period:** | 30 seconds |
| **Cool-down:** | Slow walking for 5 minutes followed by stretching |
| **Workout tips:** | * Because this program contains three sets of two chest exercises listed in order, you may need to readjust the load that you are using in exercise 2 to complete three back-to-back sets. |

## WORKOUT 3

| | |
|---|---|
| **Total time:** | 1 hour, 26 minutes |
| **Weeks:** | 5 and 6 |
| **Days of the week:** | Three nonconsecutive days |
| **Warm-up:** | Easy jogging or rope skipping for 5 minutes followed by stretching |
| **Exercises:** | 56 minutes |

|  |  |  |  | Choose 1 exercise per row | | |
|---|---|---|---|---|---|---|
| # | Muscle group | Reps | Sets | Barbell | Machine | Alternative |
| 1 | Chest | 12-15 | 4* | Bench press | Chest press | Bench press (DB) |
| 2 | Chest | 12-15 | 3 | Incline bench press | Pec deck | Chest fly (DB) |
| 3 | Back | 12-15 | 4* | Bent-over row | Seated row | One-arm row (DB) |
| 4 | Shoulders | 12-15 | 4* | Standing press | Shoulder press | Lateral raise (DB) |
| 5 | Back | 12-15 | 3 | N/A | Lat pulldown | Double bent-over row (KB) |
| 6 | Back of arm | 12-15 | 4* | Lying triceps extension | Triceps pushdown | Overhead triceps extension (DB) |
| 7 | Front of arm | 12-15 | 4* | Biceps curl | Low-pulley curl | Biceps curl (DB) |
| 8 | Thighs | 12-15 | 4* | Lunge | Leg press | Squat (DB) |
| 9 | Core | 15-25 | 4* | Good morning | Abdominal crunch | Sit-up (BW) |
| 10 | Calf | 12-15 | 3 | Standing heel raise | Seated heel raise | One-leg standing heel raise (DB) |

| | |
|---|---|
| **Rest period:** | 30 seconds |
| **Cool-down:** | Slow walking for 5 minutes followed by stretching |
| **Workout tips:** | * As you begin performing four sets in these exercises, you may have to decrease the load slightly (5-10 pounds, or ~2.5-5 kg, for exercises 1, 3, 4, and 6 through 9 and 10-15 pounds, or ~5-7 kg, for exercise 8) to allow you to complete all four sets successfully. |

## WORKOUT 1

| | |
|---|---|
| **Total time:** | 1 hour, 13 minutes |
| **Weeks:** | 1 and 2 |
| **Days of the week:** | Two nonconsecutive days |
| **Warm-up:** | Easy jogging or rope skipping for 5 minutes followed by stretching |
| **Upper-body exercises:** | 43 minutes |

| | | | | Choose 1 exercise per row | | |
|---|---|---|---|---|---|---|
| **#** | **Muscle group** | **Reps** | **Sets** | **Barbell** | **Machine** | **Alternative** |
| 1 | Chest | 10-12 | 3 | Bench press | Chest press | Bench press (DB) |
| 2 | Chest* | 10-12 | 3 | Incline bench press | Pec deck | Chest fly (DB) |
| 3 | Back | 10-12 | 3 | Bent-over row | Seated row | One-arm row (DB) |
| 4 | Back* | 10-12 | 3 | N/A | Lat pulldown | Double bent-over row (KB) |
| 5 | Shoulders | 10-12 | 3 | Standing press | Shoulder press | Lateral raise (DB) |
| 6** | Shoulders* | 10-12 | 1 | Upright row | Lateral raise | Lateral raise (DB) |
| 7 | Front of arm | 10-12 | 3 | Biceps curl | Low-pulley curl | Biceps curl (DB) |
| 8** | Front of arm* | 10-12 | 1 | Reverse curl | Preacher curl | Hammer curl (DB) |
| 9 | Back of arm | 10-12 | 3 | Lying triceps extension | Triceps pushdown | Overhead triceps extension (DB) |
| 10** | Back of arm* | 10-12 | 1 | Seated overhead triceps extension | Triceps extension | One-arm triceps extension (RB) |

| | |
|---|---|
| **Rest period:** | 1 minute |
| **Cool-down:** | Slow walking for 5 minutes followed by stretching |
| **Workout tips:** | * Because this program contains two exercises in a row for the same muscle group, you may need to adjust the load that you are using across all sets of the exercises to complete the desired number of repetitions. |
| | ** If you just completed the Yellow Zone, note the changes made in the order of the exercises and the addition of three new exercises (6, 8, and 10). Refer to chapter 4 to determine your starting loads for new exercises and chapter 6 to learn how to perform them correctly. |

## WORKOUT 2

**Total time:** 1 hour, 6 minutes

**Weeks:** 1 and 2

**Days of the week:** Two nonconsecutive days

**Warm-up:** Easy jogging or rope skipping for 5 minutes followed by stretching

**Lower-body exercises:** 36 minutes

| | | | | | Choose 1 exercise per row | |
| --- | --- | --- | --- | --- | --- | --- |
| # | Muscle group | Reps | Sets | Barbell | Machine | Alternative |
| 1 | Thighs | 10-12 | 3 | Lunge | Leg press | Squat (DB) |
| 2 | Thighs* | 10-12 | 3 | Squat | Hip sled | Step-up (DB) |
| 3** | Thighs* | 10-12 | 1 | N/A | N/A | Front squat (KB) |
| 4 | Back of thigh | 10-12 | 3 | N/A | Leg (knee) curl | Leg curl (heel pull) (SB) |
| 5 | Front of thigh | 10-12 | 3 | N/A | Leg (knee) extension | Wall squat (SB) |
| 6 | Calf | 10-12 | 3 | Standing heel raise | Seated heel raise | One-leg standing heel raise (DB) |
| 7** | Calf* | 10-12 | 1 | Standing heel raise | Seated heel raise | One-leg standing heel raise (DB) |
| 8 | Core | 15-25 | 3 | Good morning | Abdominal crunch | Sit-up (BW) |

**Rest period:** 1 minute

**Cool-down:** Slow walking for 5 minutes followed by stretching

**Workout tips:** * Because this program contains several exercises in a row for the same muscle group, you may need to adjust the load that you are using across all sets of the exercises to complete the desired number of repetitions.

** If you just completed the Yellow Zone, note the changes made in the order of the exercises and the addition of two new exercises (3 and 7). Refer to chapter 4 to determine your starting loads for new exercises and chapter 6 to learn how to perform them correctly.

ORANGE ZONE

## WORKOUT 3

| | |
|---|---|
| **Total time:** | 1 hour, 19 minutes |
| **Weeks:** | 3 and 4 |
| **Days of the week:** | Two nonconsecutive days |
| **Warm-up:** | Easy jogging or rope skipping for 5 minutes followed by stretching |
| **Upper-body exercises:** | 49 minutes |

|  |  |  |  | Choose 1 exercise per row | | |
|---|---|---|---|---|---|---|
| **#** | **Muscle group** | **Reps** | **Sets** | **Barbell** | **Machine** | **Alternative** |
| 1 | Chest | 10-12 | 3 | Bench press | Chest press | Bench press (DB) |
| 2 | Chest* | 10-12 | 3 | Incline bench press | Pec deck | Chest fly (DB) |
| 3 | Back | 10-12 | 3 | Bent-over row | Seated row | One-arm row (DB) |
| 4 | Back* | 10-12 | 3 | N/A | Lat pulldown | Double bent-over row (KB) |
| 5 | Shoulders | 10-12 | 3 | Standing press | Shoulder press | Lateral raise (DB) |
| 6 | Shoulders* | 10-12 | 2 | Upright row | Lateral raise | Lateral raise (DB) |
| 7 | Front of arm | 10-12 | 3 | Biceps curl | Low-pulley curl | Biceps curl (DB) |
| 8 | Front of arm* | 10-12 | 2 | Reverse curl | Preacher curl | Hammer curl (DB) |
| 9 | Back of arm | 10-12 | 3 | Lying triceps extension | Triceps pushdown | Overhead triceps extension (DB) |
| 10 | Back of arm* | 10-12 | 2 | Seated overhead triceps extension | Triceps extension | One-arm triceps extension (RB) |

| | |
|---|---|
| **Rest period:** | 1 minute |
| **Cool-down:** | Slow walking for 5 minutes followed by stretching |
| **Workout tips:** | * Because this program contains sequential exercises for the same muscle group, you may need to adjust the load that you are using across all sets of the exercises to complete the desired number of repetitions in back-to-back sets. |

## WORKOUT 4

| | |
|---|---|
| **Total time:** | 1 hour, 10 minutes |
| **Weeks:** | 3 and 4 |
| **Days of the week:** | Two nonconsecutive days |
| **Warm-up:** | Easy jogging or rope skipping for 5 minutes followed by stretching |
| **Lower-body exercises:** | 40 minutes |

| | | | | | Choose 1 exercise per row | |
|---|---|---|---|---|---|---|
| **#** | **Muscle group** | **Reps** | **Sets** | **Barbell** | **Machine** | **Alternative** |
| 1 | Thighs | 10-12 | 3 | Lunge | Leg press | Squat (DB) |
| 2 | Thighs* | 10-12 | 3 | Squat | Hip sled | Step-up (DB) |
| 3 | Thighs* | 10-12 | 2 | N/A | N/A | Front squat (KB) |
| 4 | Back of thigh | 10-12 | 3 | N/A | Leg (knee) curl | Leg curl (heel pull) (SB) |
| 5 | Front of thigh | 10-12 | 3 | N/A | Leg (knee) extension | Wall squat (SB) |
| 6 | Calf | 10-12 | 3 | Standing heel raise | Seated heel raise | One-leg standing heel raise (DB) |
| 7 | Calf* | 10-12 | 2 | Standing heel raise | Seated heel raise | One-leg standing heel raise (DB) |
| 8 | Core | 15-25 | 3 | Good morning | Abdominal crunch | Sit-up (BW) |

| | |
|---|---|
| **Rest period:** | 1 minute |
| **Cool-down:** | Slow walking for 5 minutes followed by stretching |
| **Workout tips:** | * Because this program contains sequential exercises for the same muscle group, you may need to adjust the load that you are using across all sets of the exercises to complete the desired number of repetitions in back-to-back sets. |

ORANGE ZONE

## WORKOUT 5

| | |
|---|---|
| **Total time:** | 1 hour, 24 minutes |
| **Weeks:** | 5 and 6 |
| **Days of the week:** | Two nonconsecutive days |
| **Warm-up:** | Easy jogging or rope skipping for 5 minutes followed by stretching |
| **Upper-body exercises:** 54 minutes | |

| | | | | Choose 1 exercise per row | | |
|---|---|---|---|---|---|---|
| # | Muscle group | Reps | Sets | Barbell | Machine | Alternative |
| 1 | Chest | 10-12 | 3 | Bench press | Chest press | Bench press (DB) |
| 2 | Chest* | 10-12 | 3 | Incline bench press | Pec deck | Chest fly (DB) |
| 3 | Back | 10-12 | 3 | Bent-over row | Seated row | One-arm row (DB) |
| 4 | Back* | 10-12 | 3 | N/A | Lat pulldown | Double bent-over row (KB) |
| 5 | Shoulders | 10-12 | 3 | Standing press | Shoulder press | Lateral raise (DB) |
| 6 | Shoulders* | 10-12 | 3 | Upright row | Lateral raise | Lateral raise (DB) |
| 7 | Front of arm | 10-12 | 3 | Biceps curl | Low-pulley curl | Biceps curl (DB) |
| 8 | Front of arm* | 10-12 | 3 | Reverse curl | Preacher curl | Hammer curl (DB) |
| 9 | Back of arm | 10-12 | 3 | Lying triceps extension | Triceps pushdown | Overhead triceps extension (DB) |
| 10 | Back of arm* | 10-12 | 3 | Seated overhead triceps extension | Triceps extension | One-arm triceps extension (RB) |

| | |
|---|---|
| **Rest period:** | 1 minute |
| **Cool-down:** | Slow walking for 5 minutes followed by stretching |
| **Workout tips:** | * Because this program contains sequential exercises for the same muscle group, you may need to adjust the load that you are using across all sets of the exercises to complete the desired number of repetitions in three back-to-back sets. |

## WORKOUT 6

| | |
|---|---|
| **Total time:** | 1 hour, 13 minutes |
| **Weeks:** | 5 and 6 |
| **Days of the week:** | Two nonconsecutive days |
| **Warm-up:** | Easy jogging or rope skipping for 5 minutes followed by stretching |
| **Lower-body exercises:** | 43 minutes |

|  |  |  |  | Choose 1 exercise per row | | |
|---|---|---|---|---|---|---|
| **#** | **Muscle group** | **Reps** | **Sets** | **Barbell** | **Machine** | **Alternative** |
| 1 | Thighs | 10-12 | 3 | Lunge | Leg press | Squat (DB) |
| 2 | Thighs* | 10-12 | 3 | Squat | Hip sled | Step-up (DB) |
| 3 | Thighs* | 10-12 | 3 | N/A | N/A | Front squat (KB) |
| 4 | Back of thigh | 10-12 | 3 | N/A | Leg (knee) curl | Leg curl (heel pull) (SB) |
| 5 | Front of thigh | 10-12 | 3 | N/A | Leg (knee) extension | Wall squat (SB) |
| 6 | Calf | 10-12 | 3 | Standing heel raise | Seated heel raise | One-leg standing heel raise (DB) |
| 7 | Calf* | 10-12 | 3 | Standing heel raise | Seated heel raise | One-leg standing heel raise (DB) |
| 8 | Core | 15-25 | 3 | Good morning | Abdominal crunch | Sit-up (BW) |

| | |
|---|---|
| **Rest period:** | 1 minute |
| **Cool-down:** | Slow walking for 5 minutes followed by stretching |
| **Workout tips:** | * Because this program contains sequential exercises for the same muscle group, you may need to adjust the load that you are using across all sets of the exercises to complete the desired number of repetitions in three back-to-back sets. |

ORANGE ZONE

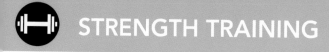
## WORKOUT 1

| | |
|---|---|
| **Total time:** | 1 hour, 21 minutes |
| **Weeks:** | 1 and 2 |
| **Days of the week:** | Two nonconsecutive days |
| **Warm-up:** | Easy jogging or rope skipping for 5 minutes followed by stretching. Before performing your first set of exercises 1 and 4, do one warm-up set of 8 to 10 repetitions with half to three-quarters of the load that you typically use for that exercise. Rest 1 to 2 minutes before starting your scheduled sets. |

**Upper-body exercises:** 51 minutes

| | | | | Choose 1 exercise per row | | |
|---|---|---|---|---|---|---|
| **#** | **Muscle group** | **Reps** | **Sets** | **Barbell** | **Machine** | **Alternative** |
| 1 | Chest | 6-8 | 4* | Bench press | Chest press | Bench press (DB) |
| 2 | Chest | 10-12 | 3 | Incline bench press | Pec deck | Chest fly (DB) |
| 3 | Back | 10-12 | 3 | Bent-over row | Seated row | One-arm row (DB) |
| 4 | Shoulders | 6-8 | 4* | Standing press | Shoulder press | Lateral raise (DB) |
| 5 | Back | 10-12 | 3 | N/A | Lat pulldown | Double bent-over row (KB) |
| 6 | Back of arm | 10-12 | 3 | Lying triceps extension | Triceps pushdown | Triceps kickback (DB) |
| 7 | Front of arm | 10-12 | 3 | Biceps curl | Low-pulley curl | Biceps curl (DB) |

| | |
|---|---|
| **Rest period:** | 2 minutes for exercises 1 and 4; 1 minute for all others |
| **Cool-down:** | Slow walking for 5 minutes followed by stretching |
| **Workout tips:** | * As you begin performing four sets in exercises 1 and 4, you may have to decrease the load by 5 pounds (~2.5 kg) to complete all four sets. |

## WORKOUT 2

| | |
|---|---|
| **Total time:** | 1 hour, 8 minutes |
| **Weeks:** | 1 and 2 |
| **Days of the week:** | Two nonconsecutive days |
| **Warm-up:** | Easy jogging or rope skipping for 5 minutes followed by stretching. Before performing your first set of exercise 1, do one warm-up set of 8 to 10 repetitions with half to three-quarters of the load that you typically use for that exercise. Rest 1 to 2 minutes before starting your scheduled sets. |

**Lower-body exercises:** 38 minutes

| | | | | Choose 1 exercise per row | | |
|---|---|---|---|---|---|---|
| **#** | **Muscle group** | **Reps** | **Sets** | **Barbell** | **Machine** | **Alternative** |
| 1 | Thighs | 6-8 | 4* | Lunge | Leg press | Squat (DB) |
| 2 | Thighs | 8-10 | 3 | Squat | Hip sled | Step-up (DB) |
| 3 | Back of thigh | 10-12 | 3 | N/A | Leg (knee) curl | Leg curl (heel pull) (SB) |
| 4 | Front of thigh | 10-12 | 3 | N/A | Leg (knee) extension | Wall squat (SB) |
| 5 | Calf | 10-12 | 3 | Standing heel raise | Seated heel raise | One-leg standing heel raise (DB) |
| 6 | Core | 15-25 | 3 | Good morning | Abdominal crunch | Sit-up (BW) |

| | |
|---|---|
| **Rest period:** | 2 minutes for exercise 1; 1 minute for all others |
| **Cool-down:** | Slow walking for 5 minutes followed by stretching |
| **Workout tips:** | * As you begin performing four sets in exercise 1, you may have to decrease the load by 10 pounds (~5 kg) to complete all four sets. |

ORANGE ZONE

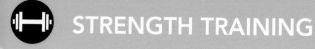

## WORKOUT 3

| | |
|---|---|
| **Total time:** | 1 hour, 30 minutes |
| **Weeks:** | 3 and 4 |
| **Days of the week:** | Two nonconsecutive days |
| **Warm-up:** | Easy jogging or rope skipping for 5 minutes followed by stretching. Before performing your first set of exercises 1 and 4, do two warm-up sets of 8 to 10 and 4 to 6 repetitions with half and three-quarters, respectively, of the load that you typically use for that exercise. Rest 1 to 3 minutes before starting your scheduled sets. |

**Upper-body exercises:** 1 hour

| | | | | Choose 1 exercise per row | | |
|---|---|---|---|---|---|---|
| # | Muscle group | Reps | Sets | Barbell | Machine | Alternative |
| 1** | Chest | 4-6* | 3 | Bench press | Chest press | Bench press (DB) |
| 2 | Chest | 10-12 | 3 | Incline bench press | Pec deck | Chest fly (DB) |
| 3 | Back | 10-12 | 3 | Bent-over row | Seated row | One-arm row (DB) |
| 4** | Shoulders | 4-6* | 3 | Standing press | Shoulder press | Lateral raise (DB) |
| 5 | Back | 10-12 | 3 | N/A | Lat pulldown | Double bent-over row (KB) |
| 6 | Back of arm | 10-12 | 3 | Lying triceps extension | Triceps pushdown | Triceps kickback (DB) |
| 7 | Front of arm | 10-12 | 3 | Biceps curl | Low-pulley curl | Biceps curl (DB) |

| | |
|---|---|
| **Rest period:** | 3 minutes for exercises 1 and 4**; 1 minute for all others |
| **Cool-down:** | Slow walking for 5 minutes followed by stretching |
| **Workout tips:** | * In exercises 1 and 4 you will perform 4 to 6 repetitions. To do this, add 5 to 10 pounds (~2.5-5 kg) to the loads from workout 1 of this zone or consult chapter 4 for a more specific method for determining new loads. |
| | ** Notice that the heavier sets of 4 to 6 repetitions require more rest between sets and a spotter for the barbell and dumbbell versions of exercises 1 and 4. |

## WORKOUT 4

| | |
|---|---|
| **Total time:** | 1 hour, 12 minutes |
| **Weeks:** | 3 and 4 |
| **Days of the week:** | Two nonconsecutive days |
| **Warm-up:** | Easy jogging or rope skipping for 5 minutes followed by stretching. Before performing your first set of exercise 1, do two warm-up sets of 8 to 10 and 4 to 6 repetitions with half and three-quarters, respectively, of the load that you typically use for that exercise. Rest 1 to 3 minutes before starting your scheduled sets. |
| **Lower-body exercises:** | 42 minutes |

|  |  |  |  | Choose 1 exercise per row | | |
|---|---|---|---|---|---|---|
| # | Muscle group | Reps | Sets | Barbell | Machine | Alternative |
| 1** | Thighs | 4-6* | 3 | Lunge | Leg press | Squat (DB) |
| 2** | Thighs | 8-10 | 3 | Squat | Hip sled | Step-up (DB) |
| 3 | Back of thigh | 10-12 | 3 | N/A | Leg (knee) curl | Leg curl (heel pull) (SB) |
| 4 | Front of thigh | 10-12 | 3 | N/A | Leg (knee) extension | Wall squat (SB) |
| 5 | Calf | 10-12 | 3 | Standing heel raise | Seated heel raise | One-leg standing heel raise (DB) |
| 6 | Core | 15-25 | 3 | Good morning | Abdominal crunch | Sit-up (BW) |

| | |
|---|---|
| **Rest period:** | 3 minutes for exercise 1**; 1 minute for all others |
| **Cool-down:** | Slow walking for 5 minutes followed by stretching |
| **Workout tips:** | * In exercise 1 you will perform 4 to 6 repetitions. To do this, add 10 to 20 pounds (~5-10 kg) to the loads from workout 2 of this zone or consult chapter 4 for a more specific method for determining new loads. |
| | ** Notice that the heavier sets of 4 to 6 repetitions require more rest between sets and a spotter for the barbell and dumbbell versions of exercises 1 and 2. |

ORANGE ZONE

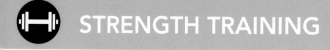

## WORKOUT 5

| | |
|---|---|
| **Total time:** | 1 hour, 34 minutes |
| **Weeks:** | 5 and 6 |
| **Days of the week:** | Two nonconsecutive days |
| **Warm-up:** | Easy jogging or rope skipping for 5 minutes followed by stretching. Before performing your first set of exercises 1 and 4, do two warm-up sets of 8 to 10 and 4 to 6 repetitions with half and three-quarters, respectively, of the load that you typically use for that exercise. Rest 1 to 3 minutes before starting your scheduled sets. |
| **Upper-body exercises:** | 1 hour, 4 minutes |

| | | | | Choose 1 exercise per row | | |
|---|---|---|---|---|---|---|
| **#** | **Muscle group** | **Reps** | **Sets** | **Barbell** | **Machine** | **Alternative** |
| 1 | Chest | 4-6 | 4* | Bench press | Chest press | Bench press (DB) |
| 2 | Chest | 10-12 | 3 | Incline bench press | Pec deck | Chest fly (DB) |
| 3 | Back | 10-12 | 3 | Bent-over row | Seated row | One-arm row (DB) |
| 4 | Shoulders | 4-6 | 4* | Standing press | Shoulder press | Lateral raise (DB) |
| 5 | Back | 10-12 | 3 | N/A | Lat pulldown | Double bent-over row (KB) |
| 6 | Back of arm | 10-12 | 3 | Lying triceps extension | Triceps pushdown | Triceps kickback (DB) |
| 7 | Front of arm | 10-12 | 3 | Biceps curl | Low-pulley curl | Biceps curl (DB) |

| | |
|---|---|
| **Rest period:** | 3 minutes for exercises 1 and 4; 1 minute for all others |
| **Cool-down:** | Slow walking for 5 minutes followed by stretching |
| **Workout tips:** | * As you begin performing four sets in exercises 1 and 4, you may have to decrease the load by 5 pounds (~2.5 kg) to complete all four sets. |

## WORKOUT 6

| | |
|---|---|
| **Total time:** | 1 hour, 15 minutes |
| **Weeks:** | 5 and 6 |
| **Days of the week:** | Two nonconsecutive days |
| **Warm-up:** | Easy jogging or rope skipping for 5 minutes followed by stretching. Before performing your first set of exercise 1, do two warm-up sets of 8 to 10 and 4 to 6 repetitions with half and three-quarters, respectively, of the load that you typically use for that exercise. Rest 1 to 3 minutes before starting your scheduled sets. |

**Lower-body exercises:** 45 minutes

| | | | | Choose 1 exercise per row | | |
|---|---|---|---|---|---|---|
| # | Muscle group | Reps | Sets | Barbell | Machine | Alternative |
| 1 | Thighs | 4-6 | 4* | Lunge | Leg press | Squat (DB) |
| 2 | Thighs | 8-10 | 3 | Squat | Hip sled | Step-up (DB) |
| 3 | Back of thigh | 10-12 | 3 | N/A | Leg (knee) curl | Leg curl (heel pull) (SB) |
| 4 | Front of thigh | 10-12 | 3 | N/A | Leg (knee) extension | Wall squat (SB) |
| 5 | Calf | 10-12 | 3 | Standing heel raise | Seated heel raise | One-leg standing heel raise (DB) |
| 6 | Core | 15-25 | 3 | Good morning | Abdominal crunch | Sit-up (BW) |

| | |
|---|---|
| **Rest period:** | 3 minutes for exercise 1, 1 minute for all others |
| **Cool-down:** | Slow walking for 5 minutes followed by stretching |
| **Workout tips:** | * As you begin performing four sets in exercise 1, you may have to decrease the load by 10 pounds (~5 kg) to complete all four sets. |

ORANGE ZONE

# 12

# Red Zone

The Red Zone is for you if you have been weight training recently on a consistent basis and scored in the high fitness classification from chapter 3, or if you completed the Orange Zone and are looking for a more advanced program. The workouts in this zone require a serious commitment to following an advanced program.

## Zone Highlights

The Red Zone covers multiple two-week workouts for each training outcome. All of the workouts in this zone have additional upper-body and lower-body exercises beyond the foundational exercises for each of the seven major muscle groups.

   If you do not have the necessary equipment or you do not feel comfortable or experienced enough to perform any of the three exercises listed for a muscle group, go to the exercise finder in chapter 6 to choose a replacement exercise for the same muscle group. Further, if you want some variety at any point in your program, you can also find a replacement exercise as long as it trains the same muscle group. Be aware, though, that your strength will not be the same because you are not used to performing the new exercise. Use the guidelines in chapter 4 to determine your starting load and then adjust that load using tables 4.10 or 4.11 to match the number of repetitions (e.g., 2-4, 8-10, or 10-12 rather than 12-15) that is listed in your zone workout table for that muscle group.

### Muscle Toning

- Weeks 1 and 2 add three more exercises—one set of 12 to 15 repetitions each for your shoulders and the front and back of thighs. To determine what loads you should use in the new exercises, refer to chapter 4.
- By the start of week 5 of this zone, you will be performing three or four sets of 12 to 15 repetitions in 13 exercises three times per week.

## Body Shaping

- Weeks 1 and 2 decrease the number of repetitions to 8 to 10 in the third set (only) of the two major upper-body exercises (a chest exercise and a shoulder exercise) and in the two major lower-body exercises (both thigh exercises). Be sure to increase the weight for these exercises (see chapter 4).
- Weeks 3 and 4 require that you perform two of the three sets in the four major exercises with a heavier weight for 8 to 10 repetitions.
- Weeks 5 and 6 add one set of 10 to 12 repetitions (now you will be doing a total of four) in the four major exercises.
- By the start of week 5 of this zone, you will be performing three or four sets of 8 to 12 repetitions in 10 upper-body and 8 lower-body exercises during four workouts per week.

## Strength Training

- For weeks 1 and 2, the MJEs now require you to perform only 2 to 4 repetitions, but you need to add weight again. Because of this change, you need to complete only three sets per MJE.
- Weeks 3 through 6 gradually add sets to the MJEs.
- By the start of week 5 of this zone, you will be performing five sets of 2 to 4 repetitions in your MJEs and three sets of 10 to 12 repetitions in five upper-body and five lower-body exercises during four workouts per week.

## WORKOUT 1

| | |
|---|---|
| **Total time:** | 1 hour, 30 minutes |
| **Weeks:** | 1 and 2 |
| **Days of the week:** | Three nonconsecutive days |
| **Warm-up:** | Easy jogging or rope skipping for 5 minutes followed by stretching |
| **Exercises:** | 1 hour |

|  |  |  |  | Choose 1 exercise per row | | |
|---|---|---|---|---|---|---|
| # | Muscle group | Reps | Sets | Barbell | Machine | Alternative |
| 1 | Chest | 12-15 | 4 | Bench press | Chest press | Bench press (DB) |
| 2 | Chest | 12-15 | 3 | Incline bench press | Pec deck | Chest fly (DB) |
| 3 | Back | 12-15 | 4 | Bent-over row | Seated row | One-arm row (DB) |
| 4 | Shoulders | 12-15 | 4 | Standing press | Shoulder press | Lateral raise (DB) |
| 5 | Back | 12-15 | 3 | N/A | Lat pulldown | Double bent-over row (KB) |
| 6* | Shoulders | 12-15 | 1** | Upright row | Lateral raise | Lateral raise (DB) |
| 7 | Back of arm | 12-15 | 4 | Lying triceps extension | Triceps pushdown | Overhead triceps extension (DB) |
| 8 | Front of arm | 12-15 | 4 | Biceps curl | Low-pulley curl | Biceps curl (DB) |
| 9 | Thighs | 12-15 | 4 | Lunge | Leg press | Squat (DB) |
| 10* | Back of thigh | 12-15 | 1** | N/A | Leg (knee) curl | Leg curl (heel pull) (SB) |
| 11* | Front of thigh | 12-15 | 1** | N/A | Leg (knee) extension | Wall squat (SB) |
| 12 | Core | 15-25 | 4 | N/A | Abdominal crunch | Sit-up (BW) |
| 13 | Calf | 12-15 | 3 | Standing heel raise | Seated heel raise | One-leg standing heel raise (DB) |

| | |
|---|---|
| **Rest period:** | 30 seconds |
| **Cool-down:** | Slow walking for 5 minutes followed by stretching |
| **Workout tips:** | * Now you are completing 13 exercises per session; to learn how to perform your new exercises, consult chapter 6. The procedure described in chapter 4 will help you determine your starting loads in these exercises. |
| | ** Be sure to perform the new exercises (6, 10, and 11) in the order listed. |

# MUSCLE TONING

## WORKOUT 2

**Total time:** 1 hour, 35 minutes

**Weeks:** 3 and 4

**Days of the week:** Three nonconsecutive days

**Warm-up:** Easy jogging or rope skipping for 5 minutes followed by stretching

**Exercises:** 1 hour, 5 minutes

| # | Muscle group | Reps | Sets | Barbell | Machine | Alternative |
|---|---|---|---|---|---|---|
| | | | | | **Choose 1 exercise per row** | |
| 1 | Chest | 12-15 | 4 | Bench press | Chest press | Bench press (DB) |
| 2 | Chest | 12-15 | 3 | Incline bench press | Pec deck | Chest fly (DB) |
| 3 | Back | 12-15 | 4 | Bent-over row | Seated row | One-arm row (DB) |
| 4 | Shoulders | 12-15 | 4 | Standing press | Shoulder press | Lateral raise (DB) |
| 5 | Back | 12-15 | 3 | N/A | Lat pulldown | Double bent-over row (KB) |
| 6 | Shoulders | 12-15 | 2* | Upright row | Lateral raise | Lateral raise (DB) |
| 7 | Back of arm | 12-15 | 4 | Lying triceps extension | Triceps pushdown | Overhead triceps extension (DB) |
| 8 | Front of arm | 12-15 | 4 | Biceps curl | Low-pulley curl | Biceps curl (DB) |
| 9 | Thighs | 12-15 | 4 | Lunge | Leg press | Squat (DB) |
| 10 | Back of thigh | 12-15 | 2* | N/A | Leg (knee) curl | Leg curl (heel pull) (SB) |
| 11 | Front of thigh | 12-15 | 2* | N/A | Leg (knee) extension | Wall squat (SB) |
| 12 | Core | 15-25 | 4 | N/A | Abdominal crunch | Sit-up (BW) |
| 13 | Calf | 12-15 | 3 | Standing heel raise | Seated heel raise | One-leg standing heel raise (DB) |

**Rest period:** 30 seconds

**Cool-down:** Slow walking for 5 minutes followed by stretching

**Workout tips:** * Be sure to perform the new exercises (6, 10, and 11) in the order listed.

## WORKOUT 3

| | |
|---|---|
| **Total time:** | 1 hour, 39 minutes |
| **Weeks:** | 5 and 6 |
| **Days of the week:** | Three nonconsecutive days |
| **Warm-up:** | Easy jogging or rope skipping for 5 minutes followed by stretching |
| **Exercises:** | 1 hour, 9 minutes |

Choose 1 exercise per row

| # | Muscle group | Reps | Sets | Barbell | Machine | Alternative |
|---|---|---|---|---|---|---|
| 1 | Chest | 12-15 | 4 | Bench press | Chest press | Bench press (DB) |
| 2 | Chest | 12-15 | 3 | Incline bench press | Pec deck | Chest fly (DB) |
| 3 | Back | 12-15 | 4 | Bent-over row | Seated row | One-arm row (DB) |
| 4 | Shoulders | 12-15 | 4 | Standing press | Shoulder press | Lateral raise (DB) |
| 5 | Back | 12-15 | 3 | N/A | Lat pulldown | Double bent-over row (KB) |
| 6 | Shoulders | 12-15 | 3* | Upright row | Lateral raise | Lateral raise (DB) |
| 7 | Back of arm | 12-15 | 4 | Lying triceps extension | Triceps pushdown | Overhead triceps extension (DB) |
| 8 | Front of arm | 12-15 | 4 | Biceps curl | Low-pulley curl | Biceps curl (DB) |
| 9 | Thighs | 12-15 | 4 | Lunge | Leg press | Squat (DB) |
| 10 | Back of thigh | 12-15 | 3* | N/A | Leg (knee) curl | Leg curl (heel pull) (SB) |
| 11 | Front of thigh | 12-15 | 3* | N/A | Leg (knee) extension | Wall squat (SB) |
| 12 | Core | 15-25 | 4 | N/A | Abdominal crunch | Sit-up (BW) |
| 13 | Calf | 12-15 | 3 | Standing heel raise | Seated heel raise | One-leg standing heel raise (DB) |

| | |
|---|---|
| **Rest period:** | 30 seconds |
| **Cool-down:** | Slow walking for 5 minutes followed by stretching |
| **Workout tips:** | * Be sure to perform the sets for exercises 6, 10, and 11 back to back and in the order listed. |

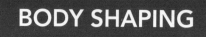

## WORKOUT 1

**Total time:** 1 hour, 24 minutes

**Weeks:** 1 and 2

**Days of the week:** Two nonconsecutive days

**Warm-up:** Easy jogging or rope skipping for 5 minutes followed by stretching

**Upper-body exercises:** 54 minutes

| | | | | Choose 1 exercise per row | | |
| --- | --- | --- | --- | --- | --- | --- |
| # | Muscle group | Reps | Sets | Barbell | Machine | Alternative |
| 1 | Chest | 10-12 8-10* | 2 1* | Bench press | Chest press | Bench press (DB) |
| 2 | Chest | 10-12 | 3 | Incline bench press | Pec deck | Chest fly (DB) |
| 3 | Back | 10-12 | 3 | Bent-over row | Seated row | One-arm row (DB) |
| 4 | Back | 10-12 | 3 | N/A | Lat pulldown | Double bent-over row (KB) |
| 5 | Shoulders | 10-12 8-10* | 2 1* | Standing press | Shoulder press | Lateral raise (DB) |
| 6 | Shoulders | 10-12 | 3 | Upright row | Lateral raise | Lateral raise (DB) |
| 7 | Front of arm | 10-12 | 3 | Biceps curl | Low-pulley curl | Biceps curl (DB) |
| 8 | Front of arm | 10-12 | 3 | Reverse curl | Preacher curl | Hammer curl (DB) |
| 9 | Back of arm | 10-12 | 3 | Lying triceps extension | Triceps pushdown | Overhead triceps extension (DB) |
| 10 | Back of arm | 10-12 | 3 | Seated overhead triceps extension | Triceps extension | One-arm triceps extension (RB) |

**Rest period:** 1 minute

**Cool-down:** Slow walking for 5 minutes followed by stretching

**Workout tips:** * When you make the change to performing sets of 8 to 10 repetitions instead of 10 to 12 repetitions, a general guideline is to add 5 to 10 pounds (~2.5-5 kg) to your upper-body exercises. At this point you have to lift the heavier weight (and perform fewer repetitions) only in the third of the three sets for exercises 1 and 5.

## WORKOUT 2

**Total time:**                  1 hour, 13 minutes

**Weeks:**                    1 and 2

**Days of the week:**   Two nonconsecutive days

**Warm-up:**             Easy jogging or rope skipping for 5 minutes followed by stretching

**Lower-body exercises:** 43 minutes

|  |  |  |  | Choose 1 exercise per row | | |
| --- | --- | --- | --- | --- | --- | --- |
| # | Muscle group | Reps | Sets | Barbell | Machine | Alternative |
| 1 | Thighs | 10-12<br>8-10* | 2<br>1* | Lunge | Leg press | Squat (DB) |
| 2 | Thighs | 10-12<br>8-10* | 2<br>1* | Squat | Hip sled | Step-up (DB) |
| 3 | Thighs | 10-12 | 3 | N/A | N/A | Front squat (KB) |
| 4 | Back of thigh | 10-12 | 3 | N/A | Leg (knee) curl | Leg curl (heel pull) (SB) |
| 5 | Front of thigh | 10-12 | 3 | N/A | Leg (knee) extension | Wall squat (SB) |
| 6 | Calf | 10-12 | 3 | Standing heel raise | Seated heel raise | One-leg standing heel raise (DB) |
| 7 | Calf | 10-12 | 3 | Standing heel raise | Seated heel raise | One-leg standing heel raise (DB) |
| 8 | Core | 15-25 | 3 | Good morning | Abdominal crunch | Sit-up (BW) |

**Rest period:**        1 minute

**Cool-down:**       Slow walking for 5 minutes followed by stretching

**Workout tips:**     * When you make the change to performing sets of 8 to 10 repetitions instead of 10 to 12 repetitions, a general guideline is to add 10 to 20 pounds (~5-10 kg) to your lower-body exercises. At this point you have to lift the heavier weight (and perform fewer repetitions) only in the third of the three sets for exercises 1 and 2.

### WORKOUT 3

| | |
|---|---|
| **Total time:** | 1 hour, 24 minutes |
| **Weeks:** | 3 and 4 |
| **Days of the week:** | Two nonconsecutive days |
| **Warm-up:** | Easy jogging or rope skipping for 5 minutes followed by stretching |
| **Upper-body exercises:** | 54 minutes |

| | | | | Choose 1 exercise per row | | |
|---|---|---|---|---|---|---|
| **#** | **Muscle group** | **Reps** | **Sets** | **Barbell** | **Machine** | **Alternative** |
| 1 | Chest | 10-12 8-10* | 1 2* | Bench press | Chest press | Bench press (DB) |
| 2 | Chest | 10-12 | 3 | Incline bench press | Pec deck | Chest fly (DB) |
| 3 | Back | 10-12 | 3 | Bent-over row | Seated row | One-arm row (DB) |
| 4 | Back | 10-12 | 3 | N/A | Lat pulldown | Double bent-over row (KB) |
| 5 | Shoulders | 10-12 8-10* | 1 2* | Standing press | Shoulder press | Lateral raise (DB) |
| 6 | Shoulders | 10-12 | 3 | Upright row | Lateral raise | Lateral raise (DB) |
| 7 | Front of arm | 10-12 | 3 | Biceps curl | Low-pulley curl | Biceps curl (DB) |
| 8 | Front of arm | 10-12 | 3 | Reverse curl | Preacher curl | Hammer curl (DB) |
| 9 | Back of arm | 10-12 | 3 | Lying triceps extension | Triceps pushdown | Overhead triceps extension (DB) |
| 10 | Back of arm | 10-12 | 3 | Seated overhead triceps extension | Triceps extension | One-arm triceps extension (RB) |

| | |
|---|---|
| **Rest period:** | 1 minute |
| **Cool-down:** | Slow walking for 5 minutes followed by stretching |
| **Workout tips:** | * In comparison to the upper-body workout 1 of this zone, this workout assigns a heavier load for the second set (in addition to the third set) of exercises 1 and 5, so you may need to adjust the load that you are using in the third set to complete 8 to 10 repetitions. |

## WORKOUT 4

| | |
|---|---|
| **Total time:** | 1 hour, 13 minutes |
| **Weeks:** | 3 and 4 |
| **Days of the week:** | Two nonconsecutive days |
| **Warm-up:** | Easy jogging or rope skipping for 5 minutes followed by stretching |
| **Lower-body exercises:** | 43 minutes |

| | | | | Choose 1 exercise per row | | |
|---|---|---|---|---|---|---|
| **#** | **Muscle group** | **Reps** | **Sets** | **Barbell** | **Machine** | **Alternative** |
| 1 | Thighs | 10-12 8-10* | 1 2* | Lunge | Leg press | Squat (DB) |
| 2 | Thighs | 10-12 8-10* | 1 2* | Squat | Hip sled | Step-up (DB) |
| 3 | Thighs | 10-12 | 3 | N/A | N/A | Front squat (KB) |
| 4 | Back of thigh | 10-12 | 3 | N/A | Leg (knee) curl | Leg curl (heel pull) (SB) |
| 5 | Front of thigh | 10-12 | 3 | N/A | Leg (knee) extension | Wall squat (SB) |
| 6 | Calf | 10-12 | 3 | Standing heel raise | Seated heel raise | One-leg standing heel raise (DB) |
| 7 | Calf | 10-12 | 3 | Standing heel raise | Seated heel raise | One-leg standing heel raise (DB) |
| 8 | Core | 15-25 | 3 | Good morning | Abdominal crunch | Sit-up (BW) |

| | |
|---|---|
| **Rest period:** | 1 minute |
| **Cool-down:** | Slow walking for 5 minutes followed by stretching |
| **Workout tips:** | * In comparison to the lower-body workout 2 of this zone, this workout assigns a heavier load for the second set (in addition to the third set) of exercises 1 and 2, so you may need to adjust the load that you are using in the third set to complete 8 to 10 repetitions. |

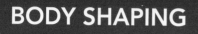

## WORKOUT 5

| | |
|---|---|
| **Total time:** | 1 hour, 27 minutes |
| **Weeks:** | 5 and 6 |
| **Days of the week:** | Two nonconsecutive days |
| **Warm-up:** | Easy jogging or rope skipping for 5 minutes followed by stretching |
| **Upper-body exercises:** | 57 minutes |

| | | | | Choose 1 exercise per row | | |
|---|---|---|---|---|---|---|
| **#** | **Muscle group** | **Reps** | **Sets** | **Barbell** | **Machine** | **Alternative** |
| 1 | Chest | 10-12<br>8-10* | 2<br>2* | Bench press | Chest press | Bench press (DB) |
| 2 | Chest | 10-12 | 3 | Incline bench press | Pec deck | Chest fly (DB) |
| 3 | Back | 10-12 | 3 | Bent-over row | Seated row | One-arm row (DB) |
| 4 | Back | 10-12 | 3 | N/A | Lat pulldown | Double bent-over row (KB) |
| 5 | Shoulders | 10-12<br>8-10* | 2<br>2* | Standing press | Shoulder press | Lateral raise (DB) |
| 6 | Shoulders | 10-12 | 3 | Upright row | Lateral raise | Lateral raise (DB) |
| 7 | Front of arm | 10-12 | 3 | Biceps curl | Low-pulley curl | Biceps curl (DB) |
| 8 | Front of arm | 10-12 | 3 | Reverse curl | Preacher curl | Hammer curl (DB) |
| 9 | Back of arm | 10-12 | 3 | Lying triceps extension | Triceps pushdown | Overhead triceps extension (DB) |
| 10 | Back of arm | 10-12 | 3 | Seated overhead triceps extension | Triceps extension | One-arm triceps extension (RB) |

| | |
|---|---|
| **Rest period:** | 1 minute |
| **Cool-down:** | Slow walking for 5 minutes followed by stretching |
| **Workout tips:** | * Because you are performing four sets of exercises 1 and 5, you may need to adjust the load that you are using in the third and fourth sets to complete 8 to 10 repetitions. |

## WORKOUT 6

| | |
|---|---|
| **Total time:** | 1 hour, 16 minutes |
| **Weeks:** | 5 and 6 |
| **Days of the week:** | Two nonconsecutive days |
| **Warm-up:** | Easy jogging or rope skipping for 5 minutes followed by stretching |
| **Lower-body exercises:** | 46 minutes |

| | | | | Choose 1 exercise per row | | |
|---|---|---|---|---|---|---|
| **#** | **Muscle group** | **Reps** | **Sets** | **Barbell** | **Machine** | **Alternative** |
| 1 | Thighs | 10-12 8-10* | 2 2* | Lunge | Leg press | Squat (DB) |
| 2 | Thighs | 10-12 8-10* | 2 2* | Squat | Hip sled | Step-up (DB) |
| 3 | Thighs | 10-12 | 3 | N/A | N/A | Front squat (KB) |
| 4 | Back of thigh | 10-12 | 3 | N/A | Leg (knee) curl | Leg curl (heel pull) (SB) |
| 5 | Front of thigh | 10-12 | 3 | N/A | Leg (knee) extension | Wall squat (SB) |
| 6 | Calf | 10-12 | 3 | Standing heel raise | Seated heel raise | One-leg standing heel raise (DB) |
| 7 | Calf | 10-12 | 3 | Standing heel raise | Seated heel raise | One-leg standing heel raise (DB) |
| 8 | Core | 15-25 | 3 | Good morning | Abdominal crunch | Sit-up (BW) |

| | |
|---|---|
| **Rest period:** | 1 minute |
| **Cool-down:** | Slow walking for 5 minutes followed by stretching |
| **Workout tips:** | * Because you are performing four sets of exercises 1 and 2, you may need to adjust the load that you are using in the third and fourth sets to complete 8 to 10 repetitions. |

## WORKOUT 1

| | |
|---|---|
| **Total time:** | 1 hour, 38 minutes |
| **Weeks:** | 1 and 2 |
| **Days of the week:** | Two nonconsecutive days |
| **Warm-up:** | Easy jogging or rope skipping for 5 minutes followed by stretching. Before performing your first set of exercises 1 and 4, do three warm-up sets of 8 to 10, 6 to 8, and 4 to 6 repetitions with one-half, two-thirds, and three-quarters, respectively, of the load that you typically use for that exercise. Rest 1 to 4 minutes before starting your scheduled sets. |
| **Upper-body exercises:** | 1 hour, 8 minutes |

Choose 1 exercise per row

| # | Muscle group | Reps | Sets | Barbell | Machine | Alternative |
|---|---|---|---|---|---|---|
| 1 | Chest | 2-4* | 3 | Bench press | Chest press | Bench press (DB) |
| 2 | Chest | 10-12 | 3 | Incline bench press | Pec deck | Chest fly (DB) |
| 3 | Back | 10-12 | 3 | Bent-over row | Seated row | One-arm row (DB) |
| 4 | Shoulders | 2-4* | 3 | Standing press | Shoulder press | Lateral raise (DB) |
| 5 | Back | 10-12 | 3 | N/A | Lat pulldown | Double bent-over row (KB) |
| 6 | Back of arm | 10-12 | 3 | Lying triceps extension | Triceps pushdown | Triceps kickback (DB) |
| 7 | Front of arm | 10-12 | 3 | Biceps curl | Low-pulley curl | Biceps curl (DB) |

| | |
|---|---|
| **Rest period:** | 4 minutes for exercises 1 and 4**; 1 minute for all others |
| **Cool-down:** | Slow walking for 5 minutes followed by stretching |
| **Workout tips:** | * In exercises 1 and 4 you will perform 2 to 4 repetitions. To do this, add 5 to 10 pounds (~2.5-5 kg) to the loads from the workout 5 of the Orange Zone or consult chapter 4 for a more specific method for determining new loads. |
| | ** Notice that the heavier sets of 2 to 4 repetitions require more rest between sets and a spotter for the barbell and dumbbell versions of exercises 1 and 4. |

## WORKOUT 2

| | |
|---|---|
| **Total time:** | 1 hour, 17 minutes |
| **Weeks:** | 1 and 2 |
| **Days of the week:** | Two nonconsecutive days |
| **Warm-up:** | Easy jogging or rope skipping for 5 minutes followed by stretching. Before performing your first set of exercise 1, do three warm-up sets of 8 to 10, 6 to 8, and 4 to 6 repetitions with one-half, two-thirds, and three-quarters, respectively, of the load that you typically use for that exercise. Rest 1 to 4 minutes before starting your scheduled sets. |

**Lower-body exercises:** 47 minutes

| | | | | Choose 1 exercise per row | | |
|---|---|---|---|---|---|---|
| **#** | **Muscle group** | **Reps** | **Sets** | **Barbell** | **Machine** | **Alternative** |
| 1 | Thighs | 2-4* | 3 | Lunge | Leg press | Squat (DB) |
| 2 | Thighs | 8-10 | 3 | Squat | Hip sled | Step-up (DB) |
| 3 | Back of thigh | 10-12 | 3 | N/A | Leg (knee) curl | Leg curl (heel pull) (SB) |
| 4 | Front of thigh | 10-12 | 3 | N/A | Leg (knee) extension | Wall squat (SB) |
| 5 | Calf | 10-12 | 3 | Standing heel raise | Seated heel raise | One-leg standing heel raise (DB) |
| 6 | Core | 15-25 | 3 | Good morning | Abdominal crunch | Sit-up (BW) |

| | |
|---|---|
| **Rest period:** | 4 minutes for exercise 1**; 1 minute for all others |
| **Cool-down:** | Slow walking for 5 minutes followed by stretching |
| **Workout tips:** | * In exercise 1 you will perform 2 to 4 repetitions. To do this, add 10 to 20 pounds (~5-10 kg) to the load from workout 6 of the Orange Zone or consult chapter 4 for a more specific method for determining new loads. |
| | ** Notice that the heavier sets of 2 to 4 repetitions require more rest between sets and a spotter for the barbell and dumbbell versions of exercises 1 and 2. |

RED ZONE

### WORKOUT 3

| | |
|---|---|
| **Total time:** | 1 hour, 46 minutes |
| **Weeks:** | 3 and 4 |
| **Days of the week:** | Two nonconsecutive days |
| **Warm-up:** | Easy jogging or rope skipping for 5 minutes followed by stretching. Before performing your first set of exercises 1 and 4, do three warm-up sets of 8 to 10, 6 to 8, and 4 to 6 repetitions with one-half, two-thirds, and three-quarters, respectively, of the load that you typically use for that exercise. Rest 1 to 4 minutes before starting your scheduled sets. |

**Upper-body exercises:** 1 hour, 16 minutes

| | | | | Choose 1 exercise per row | | |
|---|---|---|---|---|---|---|
| **#** | **Muscle group** | **Reps** | **Sets** | **Barbell** | **Machine** | **Alternative** |
| 1 | Chest | 2-4 | 4* | Bench press | Chest press | Bench press (DB) |
| 2 | Chest | 10-12 | 3 | Incline bench press | Pec deck | Chest fly (DB) |
| 3 | Back | 10-12 | 3 | Bent-over row | Seated row | One-arm row (DB) |
| 4 | Shoulders | 2-4 | 4* | Standing press | Shoulder press | Lateral raise (DB) |
| 5 | Back | 10-12 | 3 | N/A | Lat pulldown | Double bent-over row (KB) |
| 6 | Back of arm | 10-12 | 3 | Lying triceps extension | Triceps pushdown | Triceps kickback (DB) |
| 7 | Front of arm | 10-12 | 3 | Biceps curl | Low-pulley curl | Biceps curl (DB) |

| | |
|---|---|
| **Rest period:** | 4 minutes for exercises 1 and 4; 1 minute for all others |
| **Cool-down:** | Slow walking for 5 minutes followed by stretching |
| **Workout tips:** | * As you begin performing four sets in exercises 1 and 4, you may have to decrease the load by 5 pounds (~2.5 kg) to complete all four sets. |

## WORKOUT 4

| | |
|---|---|
| **Total time:** | 1 hour, 21 minutes |
| **Weeks:** | 3 and 4 |
| **Days of the week:** | Two nonconsecutive days |
| **Warm-up:** | Easy jogging or rope skipping for 5 minutes followed by stretching. Before performing your first set of exercise 1, do three warm-up sets of 8 to 10, 6 to 8, and 4 to 6 repetitions with one-half, two-thirds, and three-quarters, respectively, of the load that you typically use for that exercise. Rest 1 to 4 minutes before starting your scheduled sets. |

**Lower-body exercises:** 51 minutes

| | | | | Choose 1 exercise per row | | |
|---|---|---|---|---|---|---|
| **#** | **Muscle group** | **Reps** | **Sets** | **Barbell** | **Machine** | **Alternative** |
| 1 | Thighs | 2-4 | 4* | Lunge | Leg press | Squat (DB) |
| 2 | Thighs | 8-10 | 3 | Squat | Hip sled | Step-up (DB) |
| 3 | Back of thigh | 10-12 | 3 | N/A | Leg (knee) curl | Leg curl (heel pull) (SB) |
| 4 | Front of thigh | 10-12 | 3 | N/A | Leg (knee) extension | Wall squat (SB) |
| 5 | Calf | 10-12 | 3 | Standing heel raise | Seated heel raise | One-leg standing heel raise (DB) |
| 6 | Core | 15-25 | 3 | Good morning | Abdominal crunch | Sit-up (BW) |

| | |
|---|---|
| **Rest period:** | 4 minutes for exercise 1; 1 minute for all others |
| **Cool-down:** | Slow walking for 5 minutes followed by stretching |
| **Workout tips:** | * As you begin performing four sets in exercise 1, you may have to decrease the load by 10 pounds (~5 kg) to complete all four sets. |

## WORKOUT 5

| | |
|---|---|
| **Total time:** | 1 hour, 55 minutes |
| **Weeks:** | 5 and 6 |
| **Days of the week:** | Two nonconsecutive days |
| **Warm-up:** | Easy jogging or rope skipping for 5 minutes followed by stretching. Before performing your first set of exercises 1 and 4, do three warm-up sets of 8 to 10, 6 to 8, and 4 to 6 repetitions with one-half, two-thirds, and three-quarters, respectively, of the load that you typically use for that exercise. Rest 1 to 4 minutes before starting your scheduled sets. |
| **Upper-body exercises:** | 1 hour, 25 minutes |

| | | | | Choose 1 exercise per row | | |
|---|---|---|---|---|---|---|
| **#** | **Muscle group** | **Reps** | **Sets** | **Barbell** | **Machine** | **Alternative** |
| 1 | Chest | 2-4 | 5* | Bench press | Chest press | Bench press (DB) |
| 2 | Chest | 10-12 | 3 | Incline bench press | Pec deck | Chest fly (DB) |
| 3 | Back | 10-12 | 3 | Bent-over row | Seated row | One-arm row (DB) |
| 4 | Shoulders | 2-4 | 5* | Standing press | Shoulder press | Lateral raise (DB) |
| 5 | Back | 10-12 | 3 | N/A | Lat pulldown | Double bent-over row (KB) |
| 6 | Back of arm | 10-12 | 3 | Lying triceps extension | Triceps pushdown | Triceps kickback (DB) |
| 7 | Front of arm | 10-12 | 3 | Biceps curl | Low-pulley curl | Biceps curl (DB) |

| | |
|---|---|
| **Rest period:** | 4 minutes for exercises 1 and 4; 1 minute for all others |
| **Cool-down:** | Slow walking for 5 minutes followed by stretching |
| **Workout tips:** | * As you begin performing five sets in exercises 1 and 4, you may have to decrease the load by 5 pounds (~2.5 kg) to complete all five sets. |

## WORKOUT 6

| | |
|---|---|
| **Total time:** | 1 hour, 26 minutes |
| **Weeks:** | 5 and 6 |
| **Days of the week:** | Two nonconsecutive days |
| **Warm-up:** | Easy jogging or rope skipping for 5 minutes followed by stretching. Before performing your first set of exercise 1, do three warm-up sets of 8 to 10, 6 to 8, and 4 to 6 repetitions with one-half, two-thirds, and three-quarters, respectively, of the load that you typically use for that exercise. Rest 1 to 4 minutes before starting your scheduled sets. |

**Lower-body exercises:** 56 minutes

| | | | | Choose 1 exercise per row | | |
|---|---|---|---|---|---|---|
| # | Muscle group | Reps | Sets | Barbell | Machine | Alternative |
| 1 | Thighs | 2-4 | 5* | Lunge | Leg press | Squat (DB) |
| 2 | Thighs | 8-10 | 3 | Squat | Hip sled | Step-up (DB) |
| 3 | Back of thigh | 10-12 | 3 | N/A | Leg (knee) curl | Leg curl (heel pull) (SB) |
| 4 | Front of thigh | 10-12 | 3 | N/A | Leg (knee) extension | Wall squat (SB) |
| 5 | Calf | 10-12 | 3 | Standing heel raise | Seated heel raise | One-leg standing heel raise (DB) |
| 6 | Core | 15-25 | 3 | Good morning | Abdominal crunch | Sit-up (BW) |

| | |
|---|---|
| **Rest period:** | 4 minutes for exercise 1; 1 minute for all others |
| **Cool-down:** | Slow walking for 5 minutes followed by stretching |
| **Workout tips:** | * As you begin performing five sets in exercise 1, you may have to decrease the load by 10 pounds (~5 kg) to complete all five sets. |

# Part III

# Advanced Weight Training Programs

If you are reading this section, you have probably completed the Red Zone workouts and are ready for more! Alternatively, you may want to design your own program by calculating proper loads and choosing exercises. Either way, instructions for designing your own program are discussed in chapter 13, along with information on making program adjustments for continued improvement. Or, if like many people, you are interested in participating in a variety of activities along with weight training. If so, chapter 14 describes designing a workout plan that mixes in aerobic exercise (like walking, running, biking, or swimming) with your weight training program. If you already participate in a certain sport or activity (or want to start), go to chapter 15 to learn how to modify your current weight training program (or one found in chapters 7 through 12) to enhance your performance.

## Following a Well-Designed Program

By now, you understand the purpose of following a well-designed weight training program. Besides minimizing injury or overuse, adhering to an effective program will help you meet your training goal more quickly than haphazardly choosing exercises in the weight room. Recall that chapter 3 contains several questions to help you focus on your primary training goal. A well-designed weight training program is also based on the principle of specificity discussed in chapter 1—the crucial factor in any exercise program.

The weight training programs in chapters 14 and 15 are more advanced than those in part II because they are even more directly based on the principle of specificity. Because a primary goal of a cross-training program (chapter 14) is to improve cardiorespiratory fitness, the program includes aerobic exercise, the type of exercise most helpful in reaching that goal. Similarly, chapter 15 guides you in choosing sport-specific exercises that mimic the movements found in various sports; in doing so, it applies the principle of specificity explained in chapter 1.

# Designing Your Own Program

So you decided to design your own program! You may be in for a surprise. The process can be quite challenging because of the number of variables that you need to consider. To make this task easier, we broke down the process into six simple steps.

## Step 1: Choose Your Training Goal

As discussed in chapter 3, common weight training goals include increases in muscular endurance, size, strength, and toning and improvements in overall body shape or symmetry. Recall, however, the guidelines about training specificity described in chapter 1. For example, if you want your whole body to become bigger and stronger, the principle of specificity indicates that you choose a program geared toward developing muscular size *or* muscular strength but not both. On the other hand, you can choose different goals for different parts of the body. For example, if you are a runner you may want upper-body muscular strength but lower-body muscular endurance. What is your primary goal? Decide it now.

## Step 2: Determine Training Frequency

Before you can choose your exercises, you need to decide how many days a week you will train. Most likely, this decision is based on your personal or work schedule, how well trained you are, and how many days a week you want to commit to doing other forms of exercise (if you are cross-training, for instance).

If you are a beginner, you should perform two or three workouts a week that are spaced out evenly (e.g., Monday–Thursday or Monday–Wednesday–Friday). After you have consistently followed a weight training program for at least several months, you may want to increase the number of workouts per week to four. Again, spread out your workouts evenly throughout the week. That way you will get the recovery you need between workouts, but be careful not to give yourself too much time between the days that you train. For example, a Monday–Wednesday schedule allows too much rest between the Wednesday workout and the following week's Monday workout. When scheduling your workout days, keep in mind that no more than 72 hours should elapse between workouts that involve exercising the same muscle groups.

If you are better trained, you will be able to handle training more than three days per week, but with an odd number of days in a week, you will have to weight train on consecutive days. A *split routine* includes four or more workouts equally spread out in a week, but each workout consists of exercises that train only one part of the body (such as the upper body or the lower body). The result is that you are weight training more often but still have enough rest days between similar workouts. Many workouts in the Purple, Yellow, Orange, and Red Zones follow a split routine.

Locate the appropriate workout chart in appendix A based on the number of days that you intend to train and use it to record your workouts.

## Step 3: Select Exercises

Keep in mind the principle of specificity when deciding which body parts you will emphasize in the program and what sport or activity you are training for (see chapter 15). If your special interest is chest and arm development, then you need to include exercises that stress those muscle areas. If you have already completed some of the programs in this book, you may have found a certain exercise that you do not like; if so, don't include it in your new program.

As you select each exercise, consider what equipment you need, which ones require a spotter, and how many you can complete in the time you have available to train. Then make a list of the selected exercises and determine whether they involve free-weight barbells, machines, dumbbells, a stability ball, resistance bands, or kettlebells. In addition, if you plan to follow a split routine, you need to decide how you will group (arrange) those exercises.

## Step 4: Arrange Exercises

Decisions on arranging exercises affect the intensity of training. For example, performing the triceps extension exercise immediately before the bench press exercise will make the bench press exercise more difficult, thus increasing the intensity of the program. You can use several methods for arranging exercises, such as exercising large muscle groups first and small muscle groups last (within each half of the body; see table 13.1) or alternating upper- and lower-body exercises (table 13.2).

Another common arrangement is to alternate pushing exercises with pulling exercises. With this method, you perform a push exercise (like the bench press) after a pull exercise (like the lat pulldown) or you follow a pull exercise (like the biceps curl) with a push exercise (like the triceps pushdown). Table 13.3 provides another example of this push–pull exercise arrangement.

### Table 13.1  Arrangement of Large to Small Muscle Groups

| Exercise | Relative muscle size | Muscle group or body area |
| --- | --- | --- |
| Front squat (KB) | Large | Thigh |
| Seated heel raise | Small | Calf |
| Pec deck | Large | Chest |
| Lat pulldown | Large | Back |
| Triceps pushdown | Small | Back of arm (triceps) |
| Preacher curl | Small | Front of arm (biceps) |

Adapted, by permission, from T.R. Baechle and R.W. Earle, 2006, *Weight training: Steps to success*, 3rd ed. (Champaign, IL: Human Kinetics), 133.

### Table 13.2  Alternating Upper-Body and Lower-Body Exercises

| Exercise | Body location | Muscle group or body area |
| --- | --- | --- |
| Bench press | Upper body | Chest |
| Lunge (DB) | Lower body | Thigh |
| Bent-over row | Upper body | Back |
| Leg (knee) extension | Lower body | Front of thigh (quadriceps) |
| Lateral raise (DB) | Upper body | Shoulder |
| Leg (knee) curl | Lower body | Back of thigh (hamstrings) |

Adapted, by permission, from T.R. Baechle and B.R. Groves, 1992, *Weight training: Steps to success* (Champaign, IL: Leisure Press), 136.

### Table 13.3  Alternating Pushing Exercises and Pulling Exercises

| Exercise | Type of exercise | Muscle group or body area |
| --- | --- | --- |
| Leg press | Push | Thigh |
| Leg (knee) curl | Pull | Back of thigh (hamstrings) |
| Standing heel raise | Push | Calf |
| Twisting trunk curl | Pull | Abdomen |
| Bench press | Push | Chest |
| One-arm dumbbell row | Pull | Back |
| Shoulder press (DB) | Push | Shoulder |
| Low-pulley curl | Pull | Front of arm (biceps) |
| Triceps extension | Push | Back of arm (triceps) |

Adapted, by permission, from T.R. Baechle and R.W. Earle, 2012, *Weight training: Steps to success*, 4th ed. (Champaign, IL: Human Kinetics), 157.

No single method of ordering exercises will suit everyone; sometimes the equipment available will help make your decisions on arrangement. Whatever order you select, try to avoid taxing the same muscle group repeatedly without allowing adequate time for recovery.

After you choose a method of arrangement, add the names of the exercises you selected in step 3 to the workout chart from step 2.

## Step 5: Determine Loads, Sets, and Repetitions

This process, detailed in chapter 4, will help you set the correct loads for your new program. Start with loads lighter than you think you can lift and add weight as needed to allow you to complete the desired number of repetitions.

An exciting characteristic of weight training is that you can vary the loads, number of sets, and number of repetitions to produce the changes that you want. Table 13.4 shows you how to achieve significant strength gains by using heavier loads with fewer repetitions (1 to 8) and performing three to five sets of the most important exercises. If you want muscle toning, you need to use lighter loads with many repetitions (12 to 20) and include two or three sets of each exercise. This type of training program will also contribute to improvements in your cardiorespiratory fitness if you integrate aerobic intervals with the weight training (as presented in chapter 14). If you want body shaping, you should use moderate loads with a moderate number of repetitions (8 to 12) and perform three to six sets. Combining a body shaping weight training program with sensible eating and aerobic exercise workouts on other days of the week is an especially effective strategy for losing body fat and increasing muscle size (in men) or sculpting the body (in women), resulting in attractive changes to your body.

## Step 6: Determine Length of Rest Periods

Table 13.4 shows that you need to allow longer rest periods when training for muscular strength, moderate rest periods for body shaping programs, and short rest periods to improve muscle tone and endurance. If you are a beginner, be conservative; allow a little extra time between sets and exercises for the first several workouts so that you can gradually become accustomed to working out.

### Table 13.4 Three Outcomes of Weight Training Programs

| Outcome of training | Relative loading | Repetition range | Number of sets | Rest between sets and exercises |
| --- | --- | --- | --- | --- |
| Muscle toning | Light | 12-20 | 2-3 | 20-30 seconds |
| Body shaping | Moderate | 8-12 | 3-6 | 30-90 seconds |
| Strength training | Heavy | 1-8 | 3-5 | 2-5 minutes |

Adapted, by permission, from T.R. Baechle and R.W. Earle, 2012, *Weight training: Steps to success*, 4th ed. (Champaign, IL: Human Kinetics), 167.

## Making Continual Improvements

As your training level improves, you may want to update your program by updating one or more of the variables discussed in this chapter. This process is also called *exercise progression*. Experiment with various training approaches and find what works best for you. Although typically the more sets you perform of each exercise the more or faster you will improve, the most important factor is to train within your ability—don't overdo it! Make your training decisions carefully, based on your fitness level, experience, and training goals.

You can apply progression to your program in many ways. You may wish to perform other (or more) exercises, train more often, arrange your exercises in a different way, increase the number of sets that you perform in each exercise, lift heavier loads, or do any combination of these changes. The next section details when and how much to increase your training loads.

## When to Increase Training Loads

Soon after you determine an appropriate training load and begin using it for your program, your body will adapt to it, which means you will need to increase it to continue to make improvements. How will you know when to make those changes? There are two primary methods when determining when to increase training loads.

### Two-for-Two Rule

A conservative method is the *two-for-two rule*. When you are able to perform two (or more) repetitions beyond the goal or desired number of repetitions in the last set—and you are able to repeat that performance for two consecutive workouts—you should increase the weight in that exercise for the *next* workout.

For example, if you are supposed to perform 15 repetitions for two sets in an exercise and you become strong enough over time to complete 17 repetitions in the second (last) set for two workout days in a row (such as a Monday and the following Wednesday in a Monday–Wednesday–Friday program), you should increase the load for the *next* workout (in the example just provided, that would be on Friday of that same week).

### Set-by-Set Method

A more progressive approach when completing more than one set for an exercise involves increasing the load based on how well you perform each set (rather than for all the sets as in the two-for-two rule). If you are supposed to do three sets of an exercise, follow a 2–1–3 guideline: When you are able to perform the goal or desired number of repetitions in each set, increase the load in the second set first and complete subsequent workouts with that changed load in the second set. As soon as you are able to reach the goal repetitions in that second set, increase the load in the first set to match the load in the second set. Then, eventually, you will be able handle a load increase in the third set.

As an example, say that you can complete three sets of 10 repetitions with 100 pounds in the bench press exercise without a problem; the first change is to increase the load for the second set. Your new workout becomes 100 pounds in set 1, 110 pounds in set 2, and 100 pounds in set 3. When you are able to complete the number of goal repetitions in all three sets again, increase the load in the first set. Now you are lifting 110 pounds in set 1, 110 pounds in set 2, and 100 pounds in set 3. Over time, you will become stronger. When you can again meet the goal repetitions for all three sets, increase the load in the third set so that all three sets are at 110 pounds.

Here are the strategies for other number of sets:

- For two sets, increase the load in the first set first and then the second set.
- For four sets, increase the load in the second set first, then the first set, then the third set, and finally the fourth set.
- For five sets, increase the load in the third set first, then the second set, then the first set, then the fourth set, and finally the fifth set.

## How Much to Increase Training Loads

After following the same program for a period, you will find that lifting the original load for each exercise becomes easier. When this happens, you need to increase the loads so you can continue to make progress. It can be difficult to determine how much to increase the training loads, however.

Recall that chapter 4 explained that exercises that train larger muscles (such as the chest, shoulders, and thighs and hips) and involve two or more joints changing angles as the exercises are performed are called *multijoint exercises (MJEs)*, and exercises that isolate one muscle (or smaller groups of muscles) such as the arms, neck, and calves and involve movement at only one joint are called *single-joint exercises (SJEs)*. MJEs can safely tolerate heavier loads and larger load increases than SJEs. Thus, you have to first determine the type of exercise for which you want to increase load. Then, based on that and your training status, consult table 13.5 to see how much you should increase the load.

These loading guidelines can help you determine how much to increase the load for each exercise in the workout programs in this book, but realize that they will not work for everyone for every exercise. If the increased load is too heavy, return to the lighter load, use it in your workouts for a few more weeks, and then try to increase the load again. Often, it is a trial-and-error process, not an exact science.

### Table 13.5   Increasing Training Loads

| Training status: color zone | Description of the exercise | | Load increase |
|---|---|---|---|
| | Body area | Type | |
| Beginner: Green or Blue Zone | Upper body | MJE | 2.5-5 pounds (1-2 kg) |
| | Upper body | SJE | 1.25-2.5 pounds (0.6-1 kg) |
| | Lower body | MJE | 10-15 pounds (4-7 kg) |
| | Lower body | SJE | 5-10 pounds (2-4 kg) |
| Intermediate or advanced: Purple through Red Zones | Upper body | MJE | 5-10+ pounds (2-4+ kg) |
| | Upper body | SJE | 5-10 pounds (2-4 kg) |
| | Lower body | MJE | 15-50+ pounds (7-23+ kg) |
| | Lower body | SJE | 10-15 pounds (4-7 kg) |

Adapted, by permission, from R.W. Earle and T.R. Baechle, 2004, Resistance training program design. In *NSCA's essentials of personal training*, by National Strength and Conditioning Association, edited by R.W. Earle and T.R. Baechle (Champaign, IL: Human Kinetics), 383.

# 14

# Combining Weight Training and Aerobic Exercise

After following your weight training program for several months, you may decide that you want to add other forms of exercise to your overall program. The result of doing so is a *cross-training program*. As explained in chapter 1, in spite of the improvement in muscular strength, muscular endurance, body composition, and flexibility, the value of weight training in promoting cardiorespiratory fitness is minimal. By adding aerobic exercise to your weight training workouts, you add variety while improving your cardiorespiratory fitness. The cross-training programs that follow will help you continue to enjoy the gains made from your weight training program while improving your cardiorespiratory fitness and overall appearance.

## Cross-Training for the Muscle Toning Program

To create a cross-training program based on a muscle toning weight training program, include an aerobic exercise interval after each weight training set. The aerobic interval could consist of treadmill walking or running, stair climbing, elliptical training, stationary cycling, jogging in place, jumping rope, or any other type of aerobic exercise that you can perform near the weight training exercise stations. Initially, the length of each aerobic exercise interval should be 30 to 60 seconds. As you become better trained, the interval can be longer, the intensity of the aerobic exercise can be higher, or both.

Immediately after each weight training set, begin the aerobic interval; do not rest or pause first. If you are using an aerobic exercise machine such as a stationary bike, it is helpful to have it already set up so you can start the interval right away. Then, when the 30- to 60-second aerobic interval ends (decide in advance how long it will be), take your exercise heart rate (see the section "Determining the Intensity of the Aerobic Component" to learn how to do this).

# Cross-Training for the Body Shaping Program

To add cross-training to your body shaping program, do an aerobic workout on the days you don't do any weight training. Although the body shaping workouts will develop your muscles and shape your body, adding aerobic exercise to your overall program will increase the number of calories that you expend. The combined effect is that your body fat will decrease and your muscles will become sculpted more quickly.

You should consider your fitness level when choosing the number of aerobic exercise sessions to complete each week. If you are a beginner and follow the Green or Blue Zone workouts, add two days of aerobic exercise per week. If you are moderately trained and follow the Purple or Yellow Zone body shaping workouts, you can do aerobic exercise three days per week. If you are more advanced and are doing the Orange or Red Zone workouts, you can also add three aerobic sessions per week.

# Cross-Training for the Strength Training Program

If you are serious about developing high levels of strength, you should not add aerobic exercise to a strength training program. Because of the heavier loads required to improve muscular strength, you need to rest properly not only during the period between sets and exercises but also on days you don't do weight training as well. If you attempt to incorporate aerobic exercise into a strength training program, you will find that you may not feel recovered enough to complete the more intense weight training workouts and you may struggle through your aerobic workouts.

# Determining the Intensity of the Aerobic Component

To determine the intensity of an aerobic exercise interval or workout, use your pulse or heart rate as a guide. The faster you cycle, jog, run, walk, or swim, the higher your heart rate will be. You should monitor your heart rate during aerobic exercise so that you can determine whether you are exercising at a safe level yet exercising hard enough to improve your cardiorespiratory fitness. To determine your appropriate aerobic exercise intensity, follow these steps:

1. Determine your maximum heart rate (MHR).
   Subtract your age from 220:

$$220 - \text{your age} = \text{MHR (in beats per minute)}$$

$$220 - \underline{\hspace{2cm}} \text{(your age)} = \underline{\hspace{2cm}} \text{MHR}$$

2. Determine your target heart rate (THR).

Your heart rate should be within a range of 70 to 85 percent of your MHR. So, multiply your MHR by 0.70 and 0.85 to determine your THR range in beats per minute:

$$MHR \times 0.70 = THR \text{ (minimum)}$$

_____ (MHR) × 0.70 = _____ lowest THR

$$MHR \times 0.85 = THR \text{ (maximum)}$$

_____ (MHR) × 0.85 = _____ highest THR

For example, if you are 40 years old, your MHR is 180 beats per minute:

$$220 - 40 = 180$$

Your target heart rate range is 126 to 153 beats per minute:

$$180 \times 0.70 = 126 \text{ (minimum)}$$

$$180 \times 0.85 = 153 \text{ (maximum)}$$

For a quick assessment of your heart rate, count your pulse for 15 seconds and then multiply by 4 or refer to table 14.1. Thus, the 40-year-old's THR range based on a 15-second count would be the following:

126 beats per minute (minimum) = about 31 beats in 15 seconds

153 beats per minute (maximum) = about 38 beats in 15 seconds

### Table 14.1  Heart Rate Conversion Table

| Pulse rate (in 15 seconds) | Heart rate (per minute) | Pulse rate (in 15 seconds) | Heart rate (per minute) |
|---|---|---|---|
| 52 | 208 | 38 | 152 |
| 51 | 204 | 37 | 148 |
| 50 | 200 | 36 | 144 |
| 49 | 196 | 35 | 140 |
| 48 | 192 | 34 | 136 |
| 47 | 188 | 33 | 132 |
| 46 | 184 | 32 | 128 |
| 45 | 180 | 31 | 124 |
| 44 | 176 | 30 | 120 |
| 43 | 172 | 29 | 116 |
| 42 | 168 | 28 | 112 |
| 41 | 164 | 27 | 108 |
| 40 | 160 | 26 | 104 |
| 39 | 156 | 25 | 100 |

For example, if you felt 38 heartbeats in 15 seconds, your heart rate for 1 minute is 152.

You can feel your pulse at several places on your body. The easiest ones to find are at the radial artery on the thumb side of your wrist and at the carotid artery just below your jaw and down from your ear on your neck (see figure 14.1).

Immediately at the end of each aerobic interval or during your aerobic workout, simply look at your wristwatch or a wall clock, place your fingers at either location of your pulse, and count your heart rate for 15 seconds. Your goal is to reach but not exceed your 15-second THR range. If your pulse rate is too high, then step, pedal, jog, or jump rope more slowly. If your pulse is too low, increase your intensity.

When starting a muscle toning cross-training program, be aware that your exercise heart rate may not reach the minimum THR at the end of the aerobic interval, especially if the interval is only 30 seconds long or if it takes you time to get the aerobic machine going at the right speed. As you get in better shape, gain more familiarity with the equipment, and become accustomed to making the cross-training transition, you will be able to make the aerobic interval more demanding. The result will be improvement in cardiorespiratory fitness.

## Setting the Duration of the Aerobic Component

For the muscle toning program, the duration of your aerobic interval is the rest period between your weight training sets (approximately 30 to 60 seconds). When following a body shaping cross-training program, the duration is longer. If you are a beginner in the Green or Blue Zone, you can do 10 to 20 minutes of aerobic exercise per session. If you are moderately trained following the

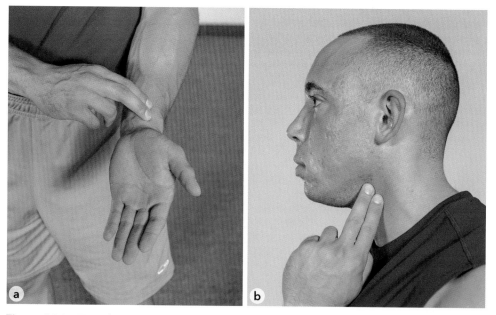

**Figure 14.1** Two places and techniques to feel your pulse: (a) at the radial artery on the thumb side of your wrist and (b) at the carotid artery on the side of your neck.

Purple or Yellow Zone workouts, you can likely handle 20 to 45 minutes. If you are advanced, you can probably complete 45 minutes or more. Be aware that these are only guidelines; for example, if you are in the Purple Zone, you do not *have* to run for 30 minutes each workout, especially if you have never run that long before. If you think that the aerobic workouts are too difficult, use a lower percentage of your MHR, shorten the length of the aerobic workout, or both. After you have become better accustomed to the aerobic workout, make increases gradually. You will be more likely to stick to your cross-training program if you enjoy it and train at an appropriate intensity and duration.

Again, as a reminder, it is not recommended that you cross-train a strength training program with aerobic exercise.

## Complete Your Cross-Training Workout Chart

If you plan to cross-train using the muscle toning program, use a cross-training workout chart in appendix A to merge aerobic activity intervals with your weight training program. Remember, all the exercises, their numbers of sets and repetitions, and the number of workouts per week remain as shown in the workout zones. Follow the two steps outlined in chapter 4 but also fill in your choice of aerobic exercise or exercises on the cross-training workout chart:

1. Determine your THR range and record it in the space at the bottom of the chart.
2. Record the name of an appropriate type of aerobic exercise in the space marked "aerobic exercise."
3. Take your heart rate immediately after completing the last aerobic interval and record it on the workout sheet.

# 15

# Weight Training to Improve Sport Performance

Many people who weight train also participate regularly in recreational or competitive sports. It is well known that weight training programs, such as those presented in chapters 7 to 12, can be modified in a way that enhances sport performance. The secret in doing so lies in the application of the principle of specificity discussed in chapter 1. The more similar the weight training exercises are to the movements of the sport, the more beneficial those exercises are in improving performance.

## Evaluate Your Sport

To apply the principle of specificity, you need to look at the primary movements involved in your sport. Observe how your whole body (especially your arms and legs) moves; if you cannot visualize those movements, have a friend videotape you or watch the sport live or on television. You are looking for repetitive motions that are part of the vital skills of the sport, frequently performed throughout the game, or both. For example, basketball involves dribbling, passing, and shooting. In each of these skills, you are repeatedly extending (straightening) your elbow against resistance (the ball) with your upper arm next to your torso (to dribble), in front of your torso (to pass), or above the shoulders (to shoot). Thus, a sport-specific weight training program for basketball should include exercises that mimic those movements.

## Choose Sport-Specific Exercises

After you identify the major skills and associated movements of your sport, the true challenge is to find weight training exercises to match them. You must choose these exercises accurately. Many exercises appear to be similar in how the body moves (like the biceps curl exercise and the triceps pushdown exercise in chapter 6). Both involve nearly the same body position and movement at the elbow, but the muscles that cause those movements are different (the biceps curl trains the muscle on the *front* of the upper arm, and the triceps extension exercise trains the muscle on the *back* of the upper arm).

Continuing the basketball example, if you observe the positions of the upper arm and the motion at the elbow, you will notice that the triceps pushdown exercise is similar to dribbling the ball, the movement of the arms in the lying triceps extension exercise is similar to what the arms do during a chest pass, and the seated overhead triceps extension exercise matches the arm movement during a free-throw shot. Your program does not need to include all three of these exercises for the triceps (unless you are a well-trained, advanced athlete); selecting even one will make your weight training program more specific to basketball.

To help with this process, look up your sport and its primary movements in appendix B. Despite the large variety of sports, most involve jumping, running, throwing, or hitting, so several common universal exercises appear throughout the table. Also, be aware that although the table includes many sport movements, not every vital or skill-related motion is listed because there are too many. The purpose of appendix B is to identify the basic sport movements and associate them with the exercises described in this book. (If you have never performed a certain exercise or need a refresher on proper technique, refer to chapter 6.)

## Insert Sport-Specific Exercises Into Your Program

After following the guidelines detailed in chapters 3 and 4 to check your weight training fitness status, choose your training goal, and determine your initial training zone, you are ready to develop a program that is more specific to your favorite sport or activity. Although a person following a general weight training program completes both steps as described in chapter 4, you will take a detour. After locating your zone workout chart in chapters 7 to 12, making a copy of the appropriate workout chart from appendix A, and choosing the days that you will train, you will replace (or add) the exercises listed for that workout with those listed for your sport in appendix B. Be sure that you exchange exercises with those that train the same muscle group or body area so that your program will still be balanced and affect your whole body. The recommendations in the "Select and Record Exercises" section of chapter 4 are still applicable; you will just be performing exercises specifically geared to improving your sport performance.

### Clarification for Green Zone Workout Programs

The exercises included in all Green Zone programs were selected because they have known factors to multiply by a person's body weight to establish starting loads (see chapter 4). To follow a Green Zone program, you may not be able to make as many sport-specific exercise substitutions. The exercises listed in appendix B do not all appear in tables 4.2 and 4.3 (load calculation tables for women and men). The best guideline is to follow the Green Zone program as listed and then modify your program to be more sport specific when you progress to Blue Zone exercises.

### Reminder About Workouts in Blue Through Red Zones

When you substitute sport-specific exercises in your program, it is possible that you will replace a MJE with a SJE (or vice versa). To minimize injury caused by overloading SJEs or to maximize the benefit of more heavily loading MJEs, be aware of which ones are MJEs and which ones are SJEs (see table 4.7). Observing this distinction will allow you to follow the guidelines in step 2 of chapter 4 to determine training loads. You will be amazed at how a program specifically designed for your sport will improve your performance.

# Appendix A

## Workout Charts for Weight Training Programs

### Two-Day-Per-Week Weight Training Program

| Zone: | | | | | Day 1 | | | Day 2 | | |
|-------|---|---|---|---|-------|---|---|-------|---|---|
| **Week #:** | | **Workout #:** | | **Date** | | | | | | |
| **#** | **Exercises** | | **Sets/ Reps** | **Set #** | **1** | **2** | **3** | **1** | **2** | **3** |
| 1 | | | | Load | | | | | | |
|  | | | | Reps | | | | | | |
| 2 | | | | Load | | | | | | |
|  | | | | Reps | | | | | | |
| 3 | | | | Load | | | | | | |
|  | | | | Reps | | | | | | |
| 4 | | | | Load | | | | | | |
|  | | | | Reps | | | | | | |
| 5 | | | | Load | | | | | | |
|  | | | | Reps | | | | | | |
| 6 | | | | Load | | | | | | |
|  | | | | Reps | | | | | | |
| 7 | | | | Load | | | | | | |
|  | | | | Reps | | | | | | |

From *Fitness Weight Training, 3rd edition* by Thomas R. Baechle and Roger W. Earle, 2014, Champaign, IL: Human Kinetics.

# Three-Day-Per-Week Weight Training Program

| Zone: | | | | Day 1 | | | | Day 2 | | | | Day 3 | | | |
|---|---|---|---|---|---|---|---|---|---|---|---|---|---|---|---|
| Week #: | Workout #: | | Date | | | | | | | | | | | | |
| # | Exercises | Sets/Reps | Set # | 1 | 2 | 3 | 4 | 1 | 2 | 3 | 4 | 1 | 2 | 3 | 4 |
| 1 | | | Load | | | | | | | | | | | | |
| | | | Reps | | | | | | | | | | | | |
| 2 | | | Load | | | | | | | | | | | | |
| | | | Reps | | | | | | | | | | | | |
| 3 | | | Load | | | | | | | | | | | | |
| | | | Reps | | | | | | | | | | | | |
| 4 | | | Load | | | | | | | | | | | | |
| | | | Reps | | | | | | | | | | | | |
| 5 | | | Load | | | | | | | | | | | | |
| | | | Reps | | | | | | | | | | | | |
| 6 | | | Load | | | | | | | | | | | | |
| | | | Reps | | | | | | | | | | | | |
| 7 | | | Load | | | | | | | | | | | | |
| | | | Reps | | | | | | | | | | | | |
| 8 | | | Load | | | | | | | | | | | | |
| | | | Reps | | | | | | | | | | | | |
| 9 | | | Load | | | | | | | | | | | | |
| | | | Reps | | | | | | | | | | | | |
| 10 | | | Load | | | | | | | | | | | | |
| | | | Reps | | | | | | | | | | | | |
| 11 | | | Load | | | | | | | | | | | | |
| | | | Reps | | | | | | | | | | | | |
| 12 | | | Load | | | | | | | | | | | | |
| | | | Reps | | | | | | | | | | | | |
| 13 | | | Load | | | | | | | | | | | | |
| | | | Reps | | | | | | | | | | | | |

From *Fitness Weight Training, 3rd edition* by Thomas R. Baechle and Roger W. Earle, 2014, Champaign, IL: Human Kinetics.

## Four-Day-Per-Week Weight Training Program

| # | Upper-Body | Sets/ Reps | Set # | Day 1 1 | 2 | 3 | 4 | Day 3 1 | 2 | 3 | 4 |
|---|---|---|---|---|---|---|---|---|---|---|---|
| **Zone:** | | | **Date** | | | | | | | | |
| 1 | | | Load | | | | | | | | |
| | | | Reps | | | | | | | | |
| 2 | | | Load | | | | | | | | |
| | | | Reps | | | | | | | | |
| 3 | | | Load | | | | | | | | |
| | | | Reps | | | | | | | | |
| 4 | | | Load | | | | | | | | |
| | | | Reps | | | | | | | | |
| 5 | | | Load | | | | | | | | |
| | | | Reps | | | | | | | | |
| 6 | | | Load | | | | | | | | |
| | | | Reps | | | | | | | | |
| 7 | | | Load | | | | | | | | |
| | | | Reps | | | | | | | | |
| 8 | | | Load | | | | | | | | |
| | | | Reps | | | | | | | | |
| 9 | | | Load | | | | | | | | |
| | | | Reps | | | | | | | | |
| 10 | | | Load | | | | | | | | |
| | | | Reps | | | | | | | | |

**Workout #:**     **Week #:**

> continued

> continued

| Zone: | | | | Day 2 | | | | Day 4 | | | |
|---|---|---|---|---|---|---|---|---|---|---|---|
| **Workout #:** | **Week #:** | | **Date** | | | | | | | | |
| **#** | **Lower-Body** | **Sets/ Reps** | **Set #** | **1** | **2** | **3** | **4** | **1** | **2** | **3** | **4** |
| 1 | | | Load | | | | | | | | |
| | | | Reps | | | | | | | | |
| 2 | | | Load | | | | | | | | |
| | | | Reps | | | | | | | | |
| 3 | | | Load | | | | | | | | |
| | | | Reps | | | | | | | | |
| 4 | | | Load | | | | | | | | |
| | | | Reps | | | | | | | | |
| 5 | | | Load | | | | | | | | |
| | | | Reps | | | | | | | | |
| 6 | | | Load | | | | | | | | |
| | | | Reps | | | | | | | | |
| 7 | | | Load | | | | | | | | |
| | | | Reps | | | | | | | | |
| 8 | | | Load | | | | | | | | |
| | | | Reps | | | | | | | | |
| 9 | | | Load | | | | | | | | |
| | | | Reps | | | | | | | | |
| 10 | | | Load | | | | | | | | |
| | | | Reps | | | | | | | | |

From *Fitness Weight Training, 3rd edition* by Thomas R. Baechle and Roger W. Earle, 2014, Champaign, IL: Human Kinetics.

## Three-Day-Per-Week Cross-Training Program

| Zone: | | | | Day 1 | | | | Day 2 | | | | Day 3 | | | |
|---|---|---|---|---|---|---|---|---|---|---|---|---|---|---|---|
| Week #: | Workout #: | | Date | | | | | | | | | | | | |
| # | Exercises | Sets/Reps | Set # | 1 | 2 | 3 | 4 | 1 | 2 | 3 | 4 | 1 | 2 | 3 | 4 |
| 1 | | | Load | | | | | | | | | | | | |
| | | | Reps | | | | | | | | | | | | |
| 2 | | | Load | | | | | | | | | | | | |
| | | | Reps | | | | | | | | | | | | |
| 3 | | | Load | | | | | | | | | | | | |
| | | | Reps | | | | | | | | | | | | |
| 4 | | | Load | | | | | | | | | | | | |
| | | | Reps | | | | | | | | | | | | |
| 5 | | | Load | | | | | | | | | | | | |
| | | | Reps | | | | | | | | | | | | |
| 6 | | | Load | | | | | | | | | | | | |
| | | | Reps | | | | | | | | | | | | |
| 7 | | | Load | | | | | | | | | | | | |
| | | | Reps | | | | | | | | | | | | |
| 8 | | | Load | | | | | | | | | | | | |
| | | | Reps | | | | | | | | | | | | |
| 9 | | | Load | | | | | | | | | | | | |
| | | | Reps | | | | | | | | | | | | |
| 10 | | | Load | | | | | | | | | | | | |
| | | | Reps | | | | | | | | | | | | |
| 11 | | | Load | | | | | | | | | | | | |
| | | | Reps | | | | | | | | | | | | |
| 12 | | | Load | | | | | | | | | | | | |
| | | | Reps | | | | | | | | | | | | |
| 13 | | | Load | | | | | | | | | | | | |
| | | | Reps | | | | | | | | | | | | |
| Date of aerobic exercise workout | | | | | | | | | | | | | | | |
| Type of aerobic exercise | | | | | | | | | | | | | | | |
| Duration of aerobic exercise | | | | | | | | | | | | | | | |
| THR range | | | | | | | | | | | | | | | |
| Actual THR | | | | | | | | | | | | | | | |

From *Fitness Weight Training, 3rd edition* by Thomas R. Baechle and Roger W. Earle, 2014, Champaign, IL: Human Kinetics.

# Four-Day-Per-Week Cross-Training Program

| Zone: | | | | Day 1 | | | | Day 3 | | | |
|---|---|---|---|---|---|---|---|---|---|---|---|
| **Workout #:** | **Week #:** | | **Date** | | | | | | | | |
| **#** | **Upper-Body** | **Sets/ Reps** | **Set #** | **1** | **2** | **3** | **4** | **1** | **2** | **3** | **4** |
| 1 | | | Load | | | | | | | | |
| | | | Reps | | | | | | | | |
| 2 | | | Load | | | | | | | | |
| | | | Reps | | | | | | | | |
| 3 | | | Load | | | | | | | | |
| | | | Reps | | | | | | | | |
| 4 | | | Load | | | | | | | | |
| | | | Reps | | | | | | | | |
| 5 | | | Load | | | | | | | | |
| | | | Reps | | | | | | | | |
| 6 | | | Load | | | | | | | | |
| | | | Reps | | | | | | | | |
| 7 | | | Load | | | | | | | | |
| | | | Reps | | | | | | | | |
| 8 | | | Load | | | | | | | | |
| | | | Reps | | | | | | | | |
| 9 | | | Load | | | | | | | | |
| | | | Reps | | | | | | | | |
| 10 | | | Load | | | | | | | | |
| | | | Reps | | | | | | | | |
| Date of aerobic exercise workout | | | | | | | | | | | |
| Type of aerobic exercise | | | | | | | | | | | |
| Duration of aerobic exercise | | | | | | | | | | | |
| THR range | | | | | | | | | | | |
| Actual THR | | | | | | | | | | | |

| Zone: | | | | | Day 2 | | | | Day 4 | | | |
|---|---|---|---|---|---|---|---|---|---|---|---|---|
| Workout #: | | Week #: | | Date | | | | | | | | |
| # | Lower-Body | | Sets/Reps | Set # | 1 | 2 | 3 | 4 | 1 | 2 | 3 | 4 |
| 1 | | | | Load | | | | | | | | |
| | | | | Reps | | | | | | | | |
| 2 | | | | Load | | | | | | | | |
| | | | | Reps | | | | | | | | |
| 3 | | | | Load | | | | | | | | |
| | | | | Reps | | | | | | | | |
| 4 | | | | Load | | | | | | | | |
| | | | | Reps | | | | | | | | |
| 5 | | | | Load | | | | | | | | |
| | | | | Reps | | | | | | | | |
| 6 | | | | Load | | | | | | | | |
| | | | | Reps | | | | | | | | |
| 7 | | | | Load | | | | | | | | |
| | | | | Reps | | | | | | | | |
| 8 | | | | Load | | | | | | | | |
| | | | | Reps | | | | | | | | |
| 9 | | | | Load | | | | | | | | |
| | | | | Reps | | | | | | | | |
| 10 | | | | Load | | | | | | | | |
| | | | | Reps | | | | | | | | |
| Date of aerobic exercise workout | | | | | | | | | | | | |
| Type of aerobic exercise | | | | | | | | | | | | |
| Duration of aerobic exercise | | | | | | | | | | | | |
| THR range | | | | | | | | | | | | |
| Actual THR | | | | | | | | | | | | |

From *Fitness Weight Training, 3rd edition* by Thomas R. Baechle and Roger W. Earle, 2014, Champaign, IL: Human Kinetics.

# Appendix B

## Sport-Specific Weight Training Exercises

| Sport | Primary movements | Sport-specific weight training exercises |
|---|---|---|
| American football, hockey, rugby | Agility type of sprinting, blocking, tackling | • Power clean, swing (KB), squat, lunge<br>• Bench press, chest press<br>• Standing press, shoulder press<br>• Biceps curl, low-pulley curl, hammer curl<br>• Seated overhead triceps extension, triceps pushdown, triceps kickback (DB) |
| Archery | Pulling | • Bent-over row, seated row, low-pulley row, double bent-over row (KB)<br>• Biceps curl, low-pulley curl, hammer curl |
| Badminton, racquetball, squash, table tennis, tennis | Racket serve, racket stroke | • Power clean, swing (KB), lunge<br>• Chest fly (DB), pec deck, bench press, chest press<br>• Lateral raise<br>• Seated overhead triceps extension, triceps pushdown, triceps kickback (DB)<br>• Abdominal crunch, extended abdominal crunch (SB), side plank (BW), twisting trunk curl (BW) |
| Baseball, softball | Throwing, batting, sprinting | • Power clean, swing (KB), squat, lunge<br>• Chest fly (DB), pec deck<br>• Lateral raise<br>• Lying triceps extension, triceps pushdown, triceps extension (CM), seated overhead triceps extension, triceps kickback (DB)<br>• Abdominal crunch, extended abdominal crunch (SB), side plank (BW), twisting trunk curl (BW) |
| Basketball | Jumping, dribbling, passing, shooting | • Power clean, swing (KB), squat, lunge, leg press, hip sled<br>• Standing press, shoulder press<br>• Bench press, chest press<br>• Lying triceps extension, triceps pushdown, seated overhead triceps extension, triceps kickback (DB)<br>• Standing heel raise, one-leg standing heel raise (DB), seated heel raise |

| Sport | Primary movements | Sport-specific weight training exercises |
|---|---|---|
| Bowling | Backswing, follow-through | • Bench press, chest press<br>• Seated overhead triceps extension, triceps push-down, triceps kickback (DB)<br>• Biceps curl, low-pulley curl, hammer curl<br>• Lunge<br>• Leg (knee) curl<br>• Leg (knee) extension |
| Boxing | Punching, blocking | • Chest fly (DB), pec deck, bench press, chest press<br>• Standing press, shoulder press<br>• Seated overhead triceps extension, triceps push-down, triceps kickback (DB) |
| Crew | Rowing (upper body), pushing (lower body) | • Power clean, swing (KB), squat, leg press, hip sled<br>• Leg (knee) extension<br>• Bent-over row, seated row, low-pulley row, double bent-over row (KB) |
| Cross-country running, cross-country skiing | Forward-type running | • Lunge<br>• Leg (knee) curl<br>• Leg (knee) extension<br>• Bent-over row, seated row, low-pulley row, double bent-over row (KB)<br>• Biceps curl, low-pulley curl, hammer curl<br>• Seated overhead triceps extension, triceps push-down, triceps kickback (DB) |
| Cycling | Pedal stroke | • Lunge<br>• Leg (knee) curl<br>• Leg (knee) extension<br>• Standing heel raise, one-leg standing heel raise (DB), seated heel raise |
| Golf | Backswing, follow-through (upper body) | • Bent-over row, seated row, low-pulley row, double bent-over row (KB)<br>• Chest fly (DB), pec deck, bench press, chest press<br>• Seated overhead triceps extension, triceps push-down, triceps kickback (DB)<br>• Abdominal crunch, extended abdominal crunch (SB), side plank (BW), twisting trunk curl (BW) |
| Gymnastics | Tumbling, rings, pommel horse, bar exercises | • Power clean, swing (KB), squat, lunge<br>• Bench press, chest press<br>• Standing press, shoulder press<br>• Lat pulldown, bent-over row, seated row, low-pulley row, double bent-over row (KB)<br>• Biceps curl, low-pulley curl, hammer curl<br>• Seated overhead triceps extension, triceps push-down, triceps kickback (DB) |
| Lacrosse, soccer | Kicking, jumping, agility-type sprinting | • Power clean, swing (KB), squat, lunge<br>• Leg (knee) curl<br>• Leg (knee) extension |

> *continued*

> *continued*

| Sport | Primary movements | Sport-specific weight training exercises |
|---|---|---|
| Martial arts | Punching, kicking, blocking | • Chest fly (DB), pec deck, bench press, chest press<br>• Standing press, shoulder press<br>• Seated overhead triceps extension, triceps push-down, triceps kickback (DB)<br>• Leg (knee) curl<br>• Leg (knee) extension |
| Skateboarding, snowboarding, surfing, waterskiing | Balancing (in a semi-squat position) | • Squat, lunge<br>• Leg (knee) curl<br>• Leg (knee) extension<br>• Standing heel raise, one-leg standing heel raise (DB), seated heel raise |
| Skating (any type) | Lunging, stroking | • Lunge, squat, leg press, hip sled<br>• Leg (knee) curl<br>• Leg (knee) extension<br>• Standing heel raise, one-leg standing heel raise (DB), seated heel raise |
| Swimming | Stroke swimming | • Lat pulldown<br>• Chest fly (DB), pec deck, bench press, chest press<br>• Lateral raise<br>• Seated overhead triceps extension, triceps push-down, triceps kickback (DB)<br>• Abdominal crunch, extended abdominal crunch (SB), side plank (BW), twisting trunk curl (BW) |
| Track and field events | Jumping, throwing, sprinting | • Power clean, swing (KB), lunge, squat<br>• Chest fly (DB), pec deck<br>• Lateral raise<br>• Seated overhead triceps extension, triceps push-down, triceps kickback (DB) |
| Volleyball | Jumping, ball blocking, ball serving, lunging | • Power clean, swing (KB), squat, lunge<br>• Standing press, shoulder press, lateral raise<br>• Seated overhead triceps extension, triceps push-down, triceps kickback (DB)<br>• Standing heel raise, one-leg standing heel raise (DB), seated heel raise |
| Walking | Walking | • Lunge<br>• Leg (knee) curl<br>• Leg (knee) extension<br>• Standing heel raise, one-leg standing heel raise (DB) |
| Wrestling | Takedown, grappling | • Power clean, swing (KB), squat<br>• Bench press, chest press<br>• Standing press, shoulder press<br>• Lat pulldown, bent-over row, seated row, double bent-over row (KB)<br>• Seated overhead triceps extension, triceps push-down, triceps kickback (DB)<br>• Biceps curl, low-pulley curl, hammer curl<br>• Abdominal crunch, extended abdominal crunch (SB), side plank (BW), twisting trunk curl (BW) |

Body weight (BW), dumbbell (DB), stability ball (SB), resistance band (RB), kettlebell (KB). Go to chapter 6 to learn the proper technique for each exercise.

# Resources

Baechle, T.R., and R.W. Earle. 2012. *Weight training: Steps to success.* 4th ed. Champaign, IL: Human Kinetics.

Baechle, T.R., and W.L. Westcott. 2010. *Fitness professional's guide to strength training older adults.* 2nd ed. Champaign, IL: Human Kinetics.

Clark, N. 2014. *Nancy Clark's sports nutrition guidebook.* 5th ed. Champaign, IL: Human Kinetics.

Faigenbaum, A., and W.L. Westcott. 2009. *Youth strength training.* Champaign, IL: Human Kinetics.

Golding, L.A., C.R. Meyers, and W.E. Sinning. 1989. *Y's way to physical fitness.* 3rd ed. Champaign, IL: Human Kinetics.

Goldenberg, L., and P. Twist, 2007. *Strength ball training.* 2nd ed. Champaign, IL: Human Kinetics.

Jeukendrup, A., and M. Gleeson. 2010. *Sport nutrition.* 2nd ed. Champaign, IL: Human Kinetics.

Kenney, W.J., J. Wilmore, and D. Costill. 2012. *Physiology of sport and exercise.* 5th ed. Champaign, IL: Human Kinetics.

McAtee, R., and J. Charland. 2014. *Facilitated stretching.* 4th ed. Champaign, IL: Human Kinetics.

National Strength and Conditioning Association. 2008. *Exercise technique manual for resistance training.* 2nd ed. Champaign, IL: Human Kinetics.

National Strength and Conditioning Association. (Baechle, T.R., and R.W. Earle, Eds.) 2008. *Essentials of strength training and conditioning.* 3rd ed. Champaign, IL: Human Kinetics.

National Strength and Conditioning Association. (Coburn, J.W., and M.H. Malek, Eds.) 2012. *NSCA's essentials of personal training.* 2nd ed. Champaign, IL: Human Kinetics.

Page, P., and T. Ellenbecker. 2011. *Strength band training.* 2nd ed. Champaign, IL: Human Kinetics.

Sharkey, B., and S. Gaskill. 2013. *Fitness and health.* 7th ed. Champaign, IL: Human Kinetics.

Westcott, W.L., and T.R. Baechle. 2007. *Strength training past 50.* 2nd ed. Champaign, IL: Human Kinetics.

# Index

# About the Authors

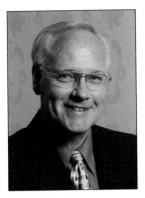

**Thomas R. Baechle,** EdD, CSCS,*D (R), NSCA-CPT,*D (R), is a professor and chair of the exercise science department at Creighton University. He is a cofounder and past president of the National Strength and Conditioning Association (NSCA), and for 20 years he was the executive director of the NSCA Certification Commission.

Baechle has received numerous awards, including the Lifetime Achievement Award from the NSCA and the Excellence in Teaching Award from Creighton University. He has more than 35 years of experience competing in and coaching weightlifting and powerlifting and presenting and teaching on these topics. Baechle has authored, coauthored, or edited 15 books, including the first and second editions of *Fitness Weight Training*, four editions of the popular *Weight Training: Steps to Success*, and three editions of *Essentials of Strength Training and Conditioning*, all published by Human Kinetics.

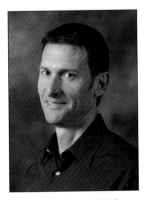

**Roger W. Earle,** MA, CSCS,*D, NSCA-CPT,*D, has over 25 years of experience as a personal fitness trainer, competitive sport conditioning coach, and behavior modification facilitator for people of all ages and fitness levels. He lectures at national and international conferences about designing personalized exercise and training programs, weight management, and exercise motivation. Previously, Earle was the associate executive director and the director of exam development for the NSCA Certification Commission, where he was responsible for reviewing and editing the CSCS and NSCA-CPT exams and writing study resources with Baechle, including coediting the first edition of *NSCA's Essentials of Personal Training* and the second and third editions of *Essentials of Strength Training and Conditioning*.

In addition, Earle coauthored the first and second editions of *Fitness Weight Training* and the third and fourth editions of *Weight Training: Steps to Success*. While at Creighton University, Earle served as the head strength and conditioning coach and was a faculty member of the exercise science and athletic training department.

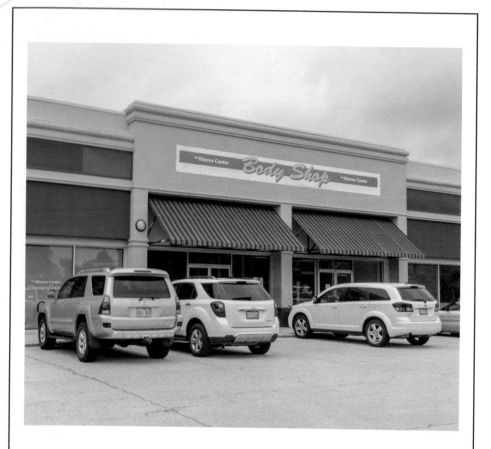

The majority of the photos appearing in this book were shot on location at the Fitness Center Body Shop in Champaign, Illinois.

The Fitness Center Body Shop
1914 Round Barn Road
Champaign, IL 61821
www.fitcen.com
(217) 356-1616